WHAT WE GUYS REALLY WANT, REALLY

A Woman's Ultimate Guide to The Male Psychology
and Sexual Behavior

By

Bryan Bruce

My Gift to You Click the Link Below

https://nowthis.life/rac/

PLEASE WRITE A REVIEW!

If this book helped you out in anyway, please help me to help others by writing a review!

https://www.amazon.com/dp/B071G7JR6H
Still, if you did not get anything new from this book or you were not impacted in some way, I would still like to hear what you have to say. Either way, I will know what am doing right or wrong and to improve in the future. I wouldn't like to take your money and not deliver. So please, take just 2 minutes to let me know what you think.

Everyone is searching for help on how to improve their lives for the better and one thing they do look for are reviews. If this book has a lot amazing reviews with great comments, they will buy the book and read it and so the ripples effects of goodness spreads. But if it doesn't have any great reviews and comments, they don't buy the book and read it.

I know this book can positively impact and help someone and you can help that person by writing your thoughts and takeaways from the book.

Additionally, I would like to read your review and hear how this book has helped you in anyway at shape or form. My plan is to print every single review and hang them on my home office wall to read for inspiration and motivation throughout the day.

Your great review helps me personally to stay focused and be able to validate all the hard work and lots of hours invested in preparing this book for you.

https://www.amazon.com/dp/B071G7JR6H
Thank you again for reading this book and all of your support, I am truly honored and grateful to have

been of help. I look forward to helping you make this year the best ever for you and your family!

Legal Disclaimer

Although the information in this book may be very helpful, it is sold with the understanding that neither the author nor the publisher is engaged in presenting specific psychological, emotional, or sexual advice. Nor is anything in this book intended to be a diagnosis, prescription, recommendation, or cure for any specific kind of psychological, emotional, or sexual problem. Each individual has unique needs and this book cannot take into account each of these differences.

https://nowthis.life/rac/

TABLE OF CONTENTS

HOW THE WRONG MEN AMONG US REVEAL THEMSELVES IN THEIR ACTIONS

Do you feel you are getting into relationships only to find out after a couple of weeks that he is not the one, he does not act as he says he is. You realize that he is the wrong guy for you and that you have made a huge mistake?

Do you feel you have been making lots of mistake in choosing the right man, always to be disappointed? Do you feel that maybe; you need to give up on men for awhile because you keep attracting the wrong men?

It's happening all the time, it doesn't matter if you live in the big city or small town. A woman meets a man she thinks is 'Mr Right' she's desperately been seeking, or a man meets his - ideal woman and it's love at first sight.

As weeks dissolve into months, she discover her dreamboat is more a nightmare, or he realize that the object of his affection is not all she appeared to be. In our fast pace world, it seems as though anything goes these days, it may be wise for both you to approach new relationships with a bit of caution.

I have researched, both men and women - there is an abundance of seemingly good catches who on closer look, turn out to be Mr. Wrong.

Yet, most you ladies subconsciously overlook fatal flaws in their lovers - for their emotional bad habits prevent them from assessing people and situations accurately... and consequently from moving on to a healthy relationship.

Red Flags to Watch Out for In Any Guy You Have Interest In
To help you distinguish between genuine jewels and worthless stones, the following are 'Red Flags' that should go up

when you are spending time with less than an ideal partner.

When he won't give you his home number:
In today's high-tech world, many people have cell phones, email, etc. However, convenience is one thing while exclusive is another.

if a man you've recently met will not give you his home telephone number or cell phone, then you have reason to suspect that he has a lots of other women or he is married.

In addition, some men like the idea of keeping track of you, but prefer that you not be able to pin down his whereabouts.

Incompatibility in basic values:
For instants, he worships Satan, she worships God. She's Catholic but he's Baptist. He has a Ph. D and enjoys intellectual discussions; She only finished grade school and has little to contribute to discussion.

He wants a lot of children and his partner to stay at home and care for them - she wants a career. Sure, it's expected that two different people will not share fully all the same values - but if most of their values are different, the relationship is in serious jeopardy.

When busy schedules leave little time for you:
Women often complain that men in their lives work all the time; Nights, weekends, holiday's etc. Or he might be an aspiring politician who attends an endless round of meetings, dinner and receptions.

Such people never have time for the family gathering - Xmas, birthday's, new years eve party. The mistakes many people make in thinking marriage will change a compulsive workaholic or would-be politician.

If you find that your love interest has a greater interest in his job or his social club, he might not be the right person for you. He's the wrong man

Emotional baggage from previous relationships:
That guy you mat seems intriguing but constantly brings up nasty tidbits about his ex-wife. Or the attractive woman who at first was like a breath of fresh air can't have a conversation without mentioning a past lover.

Get this, when you have unresolved problems from a previous relationships - it can and will carry over into the next one.

And also, when there were violations of trust in prior relationships, emotional trauma is transported into the new relationship and the carrier poses a barrier to compatibility - red flag alert. Wrong guy!

Extreme jealousy and violent behavior:
You should be very cautious about partners who are possessive, jealous and violent. Take note if your date has a bad temper and frequent angry outbursts. A red flag sign (excessive jealousy in a male partner is warning that he might become physically abusive).

Second red flag, he's paranoid all the time, the need to control, quick to get angry and constant criticism.

Men with these characteristics fit the abuser profile; Many women make excuses for violent partner - reason being that they must have done something wrong to provoke the man's actions. Early on in the relationship, it starts out with verbal abuse and afterwards it gets physical.

My advice to you; make it very clear you will not accept this kind of behavior - and even when your partner is not violent, be cautious about people who are excessively argumentative.

Note: Disagreements are to be expected, and discussions to resolve them are normal - But when nearly every disagreement escalates to an argument in 60 seconds flat, there are serious problems with this guy. Wrong guy!

The substance abuser:
A drug addict or alcoholic is the wrong choice of partner. Many substance abusers are adept at masking the severity of their problem. He may drink with you socially but also keep a bottle hidden at his bedside. Or slip into the bathroom to snort his cocaine or smoke his crack out of your presence.

Take note of your man's actions, reactions and extreme mood swings. If responses are slow, words slurred, eyes glassy - there might be a problem.

Too many nights out with the fellas or too much time with his mother:
Watch for any guy who continues to spend several nights a week out with the boys and men who spend excessive time with their family and female acquaintance while you spend time alone - obviously they fear the responsibilities of forming a solid relationship.

You should normally be turned off by men who consult with mother or friends on every aspect of the relationship, or who always tend to be on the phone with the boys when she calls or wants to be alone with him.

For example: A doctor (female) it wasn't until after she married a fireman, that she realized the control that his mother had over him. Mom would call at odd hours and insist that junior rush over and fix the (TV) or take his younger sister shopping.

Mom also had command of weekends and holidays too - after years of battling, the doctor filed for divorce and sent her Mr. Wrong home to his mother. Red flag, are you beginning to see the big picture.

Mr. Flirt:
If he constantly flirts with your sister and girlfriends, you are headed for trouble. Some men are too sociable when they take you out, they are always up in some others woman's face trying to

make you jealous.

It might be cute at first, but eventually it'll drive you batty. A man who flirts with your girlfriends will also flirt with your daughter. Stay away from such dishonest people.

Lack of communication:
It cannot be overemphasized how important communication is to a good relationship. Talking and sharing one's feelings, needs, desires, aspirations and fears are key to bonding with a potential mate.

If there are problems you must be able to talk about them to resolve them - while it might not seem like much of a problem at first, in the long run lack of communication can pose a serious barrier to intimacy.

Even when dating you should be able to communicate with your man, the inability to resolve problems in relationships is a sign of incompatibility - And also leads to boredom and nothing to talk about syndrome are (Red Flags) that you are with Mr. Wrong.

Conversations keep getting shorter and shorter, there just doesn't seem to be much to say, there are frequent long silences.

These are likely signs that your interests are so different from each other's that you have few common denominators for meaningful conversation. Or that there are few sparks of excitement to keep the relationship alive.

The control freak:
There have been many books written about this subject. Marriage counselors warned against men who must always be in control of you and the relationship. You constantly feel criticized judged and scrutinized. Or he is intent on correcting your behavior, even in front of others.

Also stay away from men who are determined to change you or whom you feel you must change. If change is needed, he might not be a suitable partner.

Don't get me wrong, we do need to change some really bad habits that we have and make compromises for a relationship.

But when he demands for change over little thing and excessively, then you need to reconsider the whole relationship.

When he has trouble keeping a job, or when his livelihood is vague and questionable:
We all know people who are involved with a partner who never seems to be able to keep a decent job. The guy will always blame 'The Black Man' or 'The White Man' or 'Racism' or 'The System' for his employment problems or whatever (black, white, pink, purple, alien, etc)

It doesn't matter. And then he would have the nerve to expect his love interests to foot the bills or make a loan to tide him over. His job doesn't have to be fancy or the salary that hefty, but a man with a steady paycheck is less likely to be a gigolo or con artist.

The gold digger:
There are some partners who expect to contribute virtually nothing to a relationship, and they may also have unfair expectations of what they should receive. We typically call these people 'gold diggers'.

They expect their romantic partners will give them more than they are willing to give others - typically they are freeloaders. You will notice the signs, when you're the only person doing all the giving! Definitely a Red Flag!

Why Wrong Men Notice You
If you've been on a dating hiatus, it's possible you have disconnected from your **feminine allure**. That means you may have lost touch with your own sensuality and your innate power of attraction.

Allure is every woman's birth right. It's your genetic heritage and nature's game plan to ensure survival of the species.

It's as simple as that. But to get the right guys to notice you here some things for you to consider-

Self-Care Builds Self-Esteem

When you start to get back into dating mode, you might find yourself spending more time on self-care. Pampering indicates that you are a woman who values her body and looks and takes good care of what she's got. This is a very good thing!

Pampering builds confidence and self esteem. Often therapists talk to clients about loving yourself first and self-care is a great step on that journey. This can range from a new hair style or make up, to new clothes, weight loss, getting in shape, etc.

How to Know When Your Allure is Working

You can tell if your allure is switched on by how others react to you. Friends, family, acquaintances and even strangers will provide the feedback to recognize that something is changing and you are on the right track.

Often the first to say something will be the women in your life, commenting on how pretty and radiant you look.

Women are nurturing and kind by nature, often acknowledging and complimenting those close to them. Next will be the men in your life who start noticing a difference in your appearance.

They'll tell you how pretty you look or that you're wearing a nice outfit and may greet you more warmly.

Some Men Are More Willing to Risk Rejection

As your self-esteem rises, so will your allure. That's when men outside your circle will start to notice you too. These will likely be the men you wish wouldn't notice you because you don't find them that attractive.

They are often a bit oblivious to your non-verbal cues (which normally keeps them away) which permits them to risk rejection

and approach you anyway.

Don't Jump to Conclusions

At this point, some women freak out, complaining that all the wrong men are attracted to them. Or wonder what's wrong that these unappealing fellows are the only ones who think they're attractive.

And as a result, they may jump to conclusions that there are no good men. Sadly, this can be the undoing of a woman's hard work to improve her allure.

Proof of Your Increasing Allure

But in truth, this is the crucial turning point. Here's a more positive way to think about the attention from less than desirable men.

They are men who find you attractive. The Universe is giving you proof of your powerful allure and the fact that your own appeal is getting stronger.

Flattery Fuels Your Allure to New Heights

If you find this happening to you, reframe the situation in your mind so that you feel flattered. You don't have to marry the flatterer, date him, or give him your number.

But you can be grateful that he has provided valuable feedback that you are attractive. Use that knowledge to fuel your self-esteem and allure to even higher levels - where you start to attract attention from the men you do want to notice you.

A Grateful Attitude Is Very Appealing

So the next time you are walking down the street and some stranger whistles, makes chauvinistic "cat calls" or pays you an unwanted compliment, in your own mind, say "Thank you." Thank you for noticing my allure. Thank you for finding me attractive.

Thank you for reminding me of and acknowledging my feminine allure. That's when you will discover that gratefulness dramatically increases your magnetism - particularly among the people you prefer to attract.

Meeting The Wrong Men? A Simple Method To Attract and Meet Mr Right

Met a lot of boring or useless men lately, and can't seem to find Mr. Right? Don't worry if you have made a few mistakes here and there, because here you will see exactly how you can use those mistakes (or even the mistakes most women make without realizing it) to attract and meet Mr. Right. So say goodbye to those other wrong matches, and say hello to this simple method to attract and meet Mr. right....

Assess yourself deeply

It may not seem like much on the surface, but you really need to start hearing yourself out if you are always attracting the wrong kinds of guys, because chances are; If you aren't meeting the right guy, it probably is your fault.

You attract what you are looking for, whether you realize it or not, and a lot of it has to do with your mental attitude.

For instance, if you think you are not too pretty and have self esteem issues....chances are, you will meet a guy who is also insecure, and also has self esteem issues which means he probably won't compliment you that often, and you will probably end up fighting a lot.

Or he will cling on too much, and act desperate, because he can't stand being alone.

Likewise, if you don't believe you can get a very successful man (you know, the smooth talker, with a 6 pack, a great sense of humor, and a solid career), who is very romantic, you probably won't get it, because your mind is closed to that option.

Start assessing how you act around us

Most women are not aware of the simple fact that men will react to them based on how they act around men in general. what this means, is that you tell a guy what to do around you, without realizing it.

But how do you do that? Well through your actions (of course). But since your actions are triggered in the mind by your thoughts and feelings this is where you basically need to assess how you act around men, and how you think in general, so you can see exactly why you have attracted the men you did in the past; and thus, stop that behavior altogether.

Failure to do so, will lead you right back to all the wrong things again, and both men and women have to do this if they truly want to meet the right person.

A simple way to begin assessing where you are going wrong or the areas of your life that need a drastic improvement is to look back at all of the arguments you've had with men in the past, by asking yourself things like:

What did you argue about?
Who started the argument, and what were they looking to get out of the argument?
Who was expecting what....and why didn't either one of you fulfill those expectations? Etc...

Once you begin to analyze your shortcomings, you can strengthen all of the best qualities within yourself and can make yourself into the woman who Mr. Right would naturally be attracted to.

WHY YOU SHOULDN'T WANT A MAN UNLESS HE WANTS THE SAME RELATIONSHIP AS YOU

Do you know what love is to a man? Do you know why men take so long to fall in love and what they think about? What are you doing wrong? Women either think they have men figured out despite being single or they believe men are complicated when they're not. Millions of women are doing it wrong.

A few things you should know about men and love:

It's a lot bigger to a man than a woman and it's not all wonderful feelings of a happy life ever after.

Love to a man means fifty years at least of one person to fight with, move to another city if her job makes them, and a minivan of three migraines. The things you should know will help you to help him.

There are going to be those days but he also needs time to see how great it could all be with a Tylenol and romantic evening with the kids at Grandma's.

Men are more rational about love and seeing the big picture before taking a leap of faith into something that no one ever knows for sure.

Remember not to pressure a man into love. A rush for love means you're trying to force something just because you want to be selfish and finally have someone to call "husband".

It's not about you so stop being a brat. Wait. If it's meant to be, it will be. One of the things you should know is that the more you push, the more you are actually pushing him away.

Take the time to just enjoy each day as it comes. Talk to each other and have long conversations about family or nothing at all but silly talk about the 2010 theory.

Get to know him in a way only a couple that has been together a while can know. Know his past and what he sees in his ideal future.

The things women should know after a few years is children, plans for thirty years from now, after retirement, and two years from now.

What Really Attracts Men Into Relationships

Would you like to know what he's thinking when he's around you? Do you know what men want from a relationship? Have you always wondered what attracts men and how to make use of that knowledge?

What is going through his mind when he's with you? Of course, it's not possible to read someone's mind. But if you can understand what many men want, you might be able to figure out your guy, and what he's thinking.

Relationships are puzzling. Sometimes people don't really understand each other no matter how long they have been together. But, men are not alien creatures either. They want many of the same things that you do.

He doesn't want to be pushed into anything. How do you react when someone tries to make you do something that you aren't ready to do, or don't want to do? He doesn't like it, either. Women sometimes seem to think that it's their job to push the guy that they want into a commitment.

But remember that men have minds, hopes, and ambitions of their own. You should be willing to let him decide for himself when he's ready to make that commitment. If he can't seem to make the leap, then he just might not be the right guy for you.

He wants a real girl. Men often have to deal with phony women. Almost every guy has been burned by a deceptive girl at some point, and many are gun-shy. If you can be yourself with him, he will instantly recognize your honesty.

If you want to know what he's thinking, you have to be willing to show who you really are around him.

You might be afraid of showing a side of yourself that's unattractive, but knowing who you are and being confident in yourself will always be more appealing than faking it. Guys like women who are down-to-earth and natural.

He wants to earn a prize. There is a reason that playing hard to get is the oldest trick in the book. It works. Anything that is difficult to obtain is perceived as much more valuable.

If you are always waiting around for him, he will sense that you are too available. If you are just a phone call away when he wants you, then you won't impress him as someone worth working for. You should not just act busy, you should be busy. Keep your independence.

He wants to be attracted to you. Yes, looks are important, and there's no point in denying or ignoring this fact. But that doesn't mean that you have to be the most beautiful girl in the world, or even in the room. It just means that physical attraction is an important part of love.

After all, you want to be with an attractive guy, don't you? However, that doesn't mean that a man has to look like Johnny Depp to appeal to you. He just has to be your type. He's looking for the same thing.

He wants to be around someone interesting. Girls who are out trying to attract attention are a dime a dozen. Women who have real substance are going to leave an impression. Men will always fall for a girl who can sustain his interest.

You will be interesting to your man if you are interesting to yourself. Stay engaged and involved with life. Keep pushing yourself to get better at the skills that interest you. Try new things regularly.

Men are different from women, but they aren't completely different. You can learn to understand what he wants from you.

DO MOST MEN WANT TO GET MARRIED AND START FAMILIES?

If there is a question that marriage counselors should start calling age old it is this one; Do men really want to get married? This is a question that women the world over ask themselves and their therapists as they seek to understand why their man just won't propose.

In truth, there is no yes or no answer to this question. Different men are surrounded by different circumstances and will therefore have varying opinions about the subject of marriage. While you cannot drag him to the alter and force him to take the vows, you can learn to understand what his fears about marriage are and help him sort them out.

Sacrifice and compromise are the two biggest characteristics of marriage. Every party has to give a little for the relationship to work. For men this is not usually a very pleasant proposition.

If they feel that their freedom is compromised by getting married, they will hold off on proposing to you for as long as they can just so they can keep their freedom to do what they want when they want to.

The best way to go about this is to help your man get a different perspective of what marriage is about. Hanging out with happily married couples has been known to help some.

Also, spending time apart every so often helps balance out his time between his world with and without you. Do not overwhelm him with your presence.

Most men want to get married but are afraid of the apparently costly affair that is marriage. Most women jinx themselves by always talking lavishly about weddings and the kind of expensive wedding they want.

If you do this you need not even ask the question do men really want to get married because he will never ask you. Do not shroud marriage in money and expenses otherwise your man will run far away from the idea no matter how much he loves you.

Men hate familiarity. The sudden realization that they have to spend the rest of their lives with one person normally hits them pretty hard. Research has also shown that men get an addictive kick out of dating many women.

Marriage does not allow for this and most therefore steer clear of marriage. This has even been pointed out as one of the reasons for infidelity in marriages. The best way to go about it is to keep the relationship exciting and fresh.

Do not get comfortable and start dressing in his clothes when you visit his apartment for the weekend. Always look sexy because this will make him want to be around you more. Men are also jealous creatures, he won't let anyone get their hands on you if you are perfect for him.

So do men really want to get married and leave the single life behind? The answer is yes. It does not matter how randy your man is, it reaches a point when he will want to settle down.

It is upon you as the woman to ease him gently into it. Do not put pressure on him to propose as this will push him away. Be an antidote for all the negative messages he hears and sees about marriage and you will soon have a rock on your finger.

What Makes a Man Want to Get Married

What makes a man want to get married? This is the question that many women wish they had an answer to. It's beyond frustrating to fall in love with a man, anticipate a life together only to realize that he just isn't interested in taking that fateful walk down the aisle to become husband and wife.

If you're in love with a man like this, don't give up on him.

Although many people will tell you that a man like this won't change, he will. Understanding what drives a man to pop the question can help you subtly guide your man towards a happily ever after future with you.

One very important answer to the question of what makes a man want to get married is security. He wants to feel that the woman he chooses to spend his life with will be there for him.

Don't try and persuade a proposal out of him by making him jealous. If he senses, even for a moment, that you may cheat on him, he'll never commit to you. He doesn't want to risk having his heart broken.

He wants to feel safe and comfortable within the relationship and the marriage. If you two are often challenging one another or if there's ongoing conflict, that's not going to help in your quest to get him to marry you.

He wants to feel that coming home each day will be a pleasant, fulfilling and peaceful experience. If you truly want a future with him you need to start working harder at showing him that you two are indeed compatible.

This may involve compromise on your part, but considering how much you value him, it's obviously worth it.

Men also crave to be committed to women who aren't standing at the ready to steal all their freedom from them. Many men are quick to say that the reason they don't want to get married is they are fearful of losing their freedom.

They still want to be able to hang out with their friends, pursue their own hobbies and have time to themselves. If you show him that you want those very same things for yourself, he'll feel even closer to you. Encourage him to go out with his friends, while you do the same.

Never ask him to change for you. If you embrace him exactly the way he is and let him know that you aren't going to monopolize his time or his life, a proposal may be in your near future.

Why Men Won't Commit

Men. Who understands them? If you've ever been confused about why men won't commit to a relationship with you, then this may help. Many women find themselves head over heels in love with a guy only to find that he doesn't seem willing to commit to a relationship.

Perhaps he's even told you he loves you, but the mention of an actual "relationship" seems to scare the Dejesus out of him.

Here are 3 reasons the man of your desire would rather remain a bachelor than commit to you-

Fear Of Giving Up His Goals And Dreams

Just like society puts pressure on women to be beautiful, it also puts pressure on men to be successful. Although success can be defined in many different ways, it's a status symbol for many men.

Women are often measured by beauty and attractiveness. Success is how men are measured in the world.

Is it fair? Of course not, but it's not likely to change any time soon, so it's important to understand if you want to understand men.

One reason men won't commit is because they feel they may have to give up their own goals and dreams to be with you. Instead of working long hours to get ahead at his job or building his own business, a man in a committed relationship is expected to spend time with his girl.

If he works too much chasing after his own idea of success, it's likely he'll get an earful about how he's never home, how he never spends time with you, is emotionally distant, etc. A serious relationship may not be a high priority at this point in his life.

Beautiful Women Abound

Many of us won't commit because we love the bachelor lifestyle. Most men fantasize about being with a variety of beautiful women throughout their life. The truth is, beautiful women abound. A man may prefer to date many women rather than committing to just one.

Some men simply aren't capable of being in a committed relationship. They either lack the self control to be loyal and faithful to one partner or they may be too emotionally withdrawn to even let anyone get that close to their heart.

Constraints On His Personal Time

A third reason why we won't commit is because we fear constraints will be put on our personal time. Men value alone time. We also highly value time with our buddies and just hanging out with the guys.

We don't want a jealous or controlling girlfriend telling us what we can and cannot do, how late we can stay out, who we can hang out with, etc.

If a man isn't ready to settle down and feels like constraints will be put on his personal time, then he may avoid having a committed relationship with anyone. It may just be a better fit for him and his lifestyle to have no strings attached.

How to Get Him to Commit Now

If your man doesn't want to get married, but you do, you have to plan your approach very carefully. Regardless of why a man says he doesn't want to get married, at some point in his life, it's highly likely that he will.

If you love him, you want the woman he marries to be you, so you need to ensure that happens. Start with stopping all marriage related talk. As a woman, you often just tell your man exactly what's on you mind, including how badly you want to get married.

If you've told him once that you'd love to be his wife, that's enough. Don't leave any hints for him and stop mentioning how lucky your friends are who are getting married. The more you push a man towards something, the more he will pull away in the opposite direction.

Just as men pull back when things become too serious for them, women should be doing the very same thing. If your man does not want to get married, don't give him free and unlimited access to you emotionally any longer. Pull back from him.

Do it carefully and subtly. Easy ways to accomplish this are to be less available and to not see him as often as you did. Stop spending the night at his place and start planning some outings with friends, without him.

Show him that you have a life outside of your time with him. Let him sense that you are starting to slip away from him. Once a man feels this, he is much more likely to rethink the whole idea of marriage. It may just spur him on to go out and buy a ring before you know it.

IS YOUR MAN A PLAYER OR DOES HE JUST NOT WANT TO BE IN A RELATIONSHIP WITH YOU?

One Woman Man Or Player? - Find Out the Truth

Is your man a player? Is he only after sex and multiple women? Are you ready to evaluate your relationship and find out the truth? There are some men out there who are in it for sex only.

They move from woman to woman and often have more than one at a time. If you have a feeling that your man might be one of these men then now is the time to evaluate your relationship.

If you want to find out the truth about your man now is the time to see whether he is a one woman man or a player.

His actions.

They say that actions speak louder than words every time because it is true. You want to look at how he acts. Each of his actions should match his words. He should stay the same.

Often players will be charming at the start of the relationship, but as time goes on they become more and more distant.

If you notice changes in his behavior then it is likely that you should step back and keep looking.

He keeps his word.

You should also take the time to check out the words that he says and the promises that he makes. A man who is interested in a meaningful relationship will strive to keep his word.

However, a player is one who will lie, make promises he doesn't keep, and you catch him in lame excuses.

You Can Contact Him.

In a strong relationship you can contact your man in many

different ways and he is consistently there. On the other hand, a player will give you his number, but there will be times that he won't be available. As time goes on it is likely that it will be harder and harder for you to get a hold of him because he will be busy.

Truth.

While you are evaluating your relationship you should make sure that you are telling the truth to yourself. You need to be open and honest with yourself if you want to find out the truth about your man.

Is He Just Playing Games With My Head?

As a woman, how good is your judgment when it comes to knowing whether a man is sincere or he is just playing you? Are you able to segregate the good guys from the users? If you are told that there's a guide to weeding them out, would you like to have that list in your hands?

If you want the guide, then go to https://nowthis.life/rac/_

He's a player if he's inattentive.

This isn't just about attention spans anymore. This is about a man who can sit there long enough to listen to what you're saying. He's also a man who looks directly at you as you speak with him.

He's a player if he says the sweetest words when you're around.

Yet you hear through the grapevine that he's been badmouthing you behind your back. These mixed signals are glaring red flags that you already have to take account of.

He's a player if his face won't even light up when he sees you.

Look at his face the moment he sees you enter the room. Does he immediately smile? Or does he only smile when you tell him that you're going to a motel after going out of the party that you're both attending?

He's a player if he's more than ready to dash off after sex.

Does this guy even speak with you after you do the deed? If he doesn't even care enough to tell you that he loves you after having sex with you, if he can't even stay to cuddle for a few minutes, then what you have with you is a worthless guy.

He's a player if he just says the things that flatter you.

But remember that there's a big difference between flattery and sincere appreciation. In order to know if he's merely flattering you, look him in the eye. He'd have to be a really good liar in order to state a lie while looking you in the eye.

He's a player if he treats you like crap.

No woman (even the bag lady!) deserves to be treated like dirt. A guy who uses you for all he can - sex, money, and attention yet is not ready to reciprocate these isn't a decent man at all.

If he doesn't find it hard to raise his voice at you - whether there's just the two of you or you are in public - then he's a man that you have to dump ASAP.

He's a player if he makes decisions on his own.

Since you're not important to him, the guy wouldn't even bother to ask for your opinion when he's on the verge of making a great decision. He will believe only on his own decisions because your opinion means very little to him.

Know The Reason Why He Doesn't Call

When you are into a guy and he suddenly is not calling you or has not attempted calling you after your first or second meeting, it will awaken all the paranoia in you. And the common reaction is you wonder why he doesn't call. Shall I call him instead?

But before you do that, you should try to weigh things first. While there is nothing wrong making the first move, it would be better if you do a little more thinking and consideration.

There are several reasons why a guy does not call. (Some of those reasons you may not even want to know anymore.)

He might be a player

It is natural for guys to make women go gaga over their phone calls. It is sort of a game for them and this is all over our genes.

There are some guys that would not like to seem desperate so they tend to hold back their desire of calling a girl; they postpone the call from a few days to a week. For them, it can diminish their masculinity and that is the greatest of their fears.

Typically, a player would just let a week pass before he calls a girl. But if after this 'grace period' you have given has expired, then maybe it is time to stop waiting for that precious call.

Don't be the desperate fallback

Now, when you have surrendered waiting for his call and he suddenly rings you and asks for another date, take this as a warning: this guy has some other priorities in life like his career maybe and he just sees you as a fallback when some of his plans or goals are not falling into the right places.

A warning he is married

If you meet a guy and you wait for weeks or days before he gives you another call, then he is probably a married man. If he is not able to give you reasonable validations as to where he has been or what he has been doing during the days or period he wasn't calling, then just be civil and find someone better; one who is more credible and not acting suspiciously.

Some other probable causes

Being busy with his job is easy to use as an alibi but not a lot of women are still buying this. You might be getting so hopeful with a guy who makes his job as an excuse to meet up with the other guys or probably even other women.

If his job requires a great deal of traveling like when he is a military guy, then this could be a valid excuse for we all know how strict the environment in the military is especially when they are out on missions.

So it is important that you know a little background about his profession. If his job gives him all the access to a phone but does not even bother give you a short call, then he is not a good candidate for a boyfriend or a husband.

WHY MOST MEN DON'T ASK FOR RELATIONSHIP HELP OR WANT TO UNDERSTAND WOMEN BETTER

Have you ever wondered why most men don't ask for relationship help when they're having problems? Maybe he's having trouble at work, financial problems, and an illness in the family etc.

Whatever the issue, a lot of men will begin to pull away from the woman in their lives thereby causing unending relationship problems when they are facing certain issues.

As a woman, you want to be there for your man when he needs you. The problem is, when a man is facing difficult times in his life he often prefers to be alone. You must not take it personally; men and women are just different.

Generally speaking, when a woman has a problem, she wants someone to listen to her. She wants to talk about the things that are bothering her. She doesn't necessarily want someone to solve the problem for her; she just wants someone to listen.

Most men are exactly the opposite. They don't want to talk about their relationship problems, they just want some time to figure things out and fix it for themselves.

That is a big reason why men don't ask for relationship help when there is problem. They just want some time to figure things out.

If you are in the beginning stages of a relationship, the man you are dating may call, text, or e-mail less often when problem arises. In a long-term relationship, or even in a marriage, your man may need some time to himself and disappear to his man cave to figure things out.

Sometimes men just need something to occupy their time for a while. A woman may think a man is wasting time when he is playing a videogame or tinkering with something in the garage, but a man who is dealing with relationship problems needs to do something that he finds relaxing and enjoyable to take his mind off things for a while.

The last thing a lot of men want to do when they are having relationship problems is to talk about their feelings.

It's important to give your man the space he needs when he is having problems communicating with you. Eventually he will figure things out and your relationship will return to normal. As a woman, it is important to understand that about your man.

If he goes into his den, garage, man cave etc. he really doesn't want you to follow him in there, trying to get him to talk about what is bothering him.

If he tells you that things between the two of you are fine and that he is just dealing with some issues, give him the space and time he needs to work things out by himself.

Is He Looking For a Relationship Or Someone To Casually Date?

Women ask me all the time, "How can I tell if a man is looking for a serious relationship, or if he just wants to casually date? What can you look for early on in dating to be able to tell so you don't waste time?"

Some men are looking for life-long partnership, some men are born wanting that - and some men are born wanting freedom. Some men are just not cut out for long-term relationships - they're just not willing to learn what they need to learn or do what it takes to "get the girl and keep her."

Different men have different capacities and abilities at different moments in time, and there are all kinds of different matches for you.

Some people are cut out for domesticity, and some people are cut out for "freedom."

The truth is, domesticity and a dangerous, "exciting" type of man don't mix very well. Domesticity by nature might seem kind of boring - it's "everyday" and it's about familiarity, which some people say eventually kills sexual attraction.

You have to work through that to build intimacy. Intimacy, in my opinion, is a way into sexual attraction.

Practically speaking, when it comes to dating, if a man isn't 100% available for the kind of relationship you're looking for - he doesn't get one second of your time, energy, or attention.

That's a requirement, because It's easy to get all wrapped up with these "exciting" men who just aren't cut out for long-term partnership.

That's why it's so important to not invest in any one man until he's offering you everything you want.

For example, if you're looking to have kids within the next couple of years and that's really important to you, you don't want to invest your time and energy into someone who "might want kids someday" or someone who says he doesn't want kids - and hope you will change his mind. That's a recipe for disappointment and **heartbreak.**

For these bigger issues, a man has to be on the same page as you for him to even qualify - and his energy has to be coming to-wards you.

If a man's energy isn't coming towards you - or if you can't feel relaxed and be yourself around him - just drop him! It's not worth your time or energy to even think about a man who's not totally crazy about you. If he's not, just forget about him and move on to the type of men who would do anything to be with you.

The key is to let men do what they're going to do, **while you lean back and just watch them** to see whether or not you're on the same page, without getting hung up on any one of them until they decide to stay - until they come across with what you're looking for in a relationship.

Dating may seem like a full-time job - and yet if what you want is a meaningful, fulfilling relationship - I believe it's totally worth the full-time job.

Why Men Pull Away and How To Understand Them

Have you ever asked yourself why men pull away? You could be in a loving, committed relationship, things are going well, you are both happy, you might even be wondering if he's the one, and then for apparently no reason at all he pulls away.

Given that everything was going so well you are likely to be confused and hurt, uncertain as to whether your relationship has any future. Hard as it may seem, there is every chance that your guy is confused as well.

If you have a relationship worth fighting for then you have to be able to understand your man, what motivates him and what scares him.

Let's start with the more pathetic reasons as to why men pull away. We should say that the following reasons by no means cover the majority of cases, but you do need to be aware of them.

The most basic is that he's not interested. It could be that all he wanted to do was have his wicked way with you and now he wants to drift on to his next conquest.

It could be the case that he has another girlfriend, or worse, but he's too much of a coward to tell you, so instead he pulls away and leaves you wondering what has happened.

And it could also be that he came to you on the rebound. he might have needed to prove to himself that he still has it, and having done so he is no longer interested in you.

It's possible that he doesn't feel compatible with you, and instead of talking things through with you, he just pulls away. In this case it's possible that you might not be a compatible couple, but before you make a judgement on that, you need to talk things through to see if there is a way forward.

There's also the problem that some men are just plain selfish, the whole universe revolves around them, and if you won't subscribe to that state of being then you are of no interest to them.

If your situation fits into any of those 4 scenarios, then please let this guy pull away as far as possible. You don't need someone like that, and you are highly unlikely to have a lasting, fulfilling relationship with an individual like that!

Right then, having dealt with the dross, we now need to look at what happens when you are in what should be a happy and fulfilling relationship. Trying to build an unreal, fantasy relationship will make men pull away.

The first thing to do is to take a look at what a relationship is, and should be. First and foremost, regardless of what either of you bring to the relationship you are two equal partners, and you have an equal responsibility for making your relationship work.

You have to be able to communicate with each other, you have to be able to share things and open up with each other.

Having a physical attraction is great, but it's communication that makes and develops a relationship, and as many couples have found, when the communication goes you no longer have a relationship.

What is probably the most important thing of all is that you have to love each other for who you are, you should never try to change each other because if you change him, will he still be the same person that you fell in love with?

You have your relationship. Can you tell if you view your relationship with rosy tinted spectacles, or do you accept your relationship for what it is.

There are far too many women who have allowed their perception of what a relationship is to be colored by what they see in the movies or what they read in books. Similarly; what you have seen and read can also color how you view your partner.

Now these perceptions may be great in an ideal world, but we don't live in an ideal world, we live in the real world. In the real world you have to accept your situation, you have to accept who you have fallen in love with, and you have to build a relationship around that.

If you are unable to accept reality and try to create some fantasy idyll you could have your guy running for the hills.

No one is to say that you can't stop him from doing things like picking his nose in public, but unless you accept who he is and your own personal situation, then will you ever be truly satisfied or happy.

And if you come across as not satisfied or happy what will your guy think, will he pull away or will he stay in your unfulfilling relationship?

You both came into this relationship with your own histories, your friends and families, your hobbies and interests, nothing can change that, and just because you are in a relationship it doesn't mean that you have to bid farewell to these integral parts of you.

One of the things that men fear is that they will lose the sense of who they are, they might be worried that they can't do guy things, that they will no longer be able to hang out with their friends, have a few beers, watch the game and just chill.

If you want your relationship to succeed then as well as being an integral part of each other's lives, you also have to be able to lead your own lives.

You cannot live in each other's pockets 24/7, doing that will not only drive you both crazy but it will stunt the growth of your relationship, and the growth of both of you as individuals. We grow as people by experiencing life.

A relationship grows when both of you can bring all of your ever-changing experiences to the table. If you can't have your own lives then your relationship will become dull and boring.

If all you ever do is share exactly the same experiences, then where is the depth of life that makes you who you are.

If he has started to pull away make sure that he understands that he doesn't have to lose his old life.

When a man starts to pull away it could be that he fears losing his individuality and everything that **"he thinks"** makes him a man. If your relationship has become too close it could be that your guy feels that you are smothering him.

If that is the case then you need to give him the opportunity to do his own thing, and just as he can go and do his own thing then so should you. Remember, everything that you did before you met made you the people who you are.

Men pull away because they don't want to lose who they are. And whilst you can't spend the time on everything that you did before meeting each other, it's healthy to have some you space.

You will develop as people, as you develop your relationship will develop, and just think of all the things that you will have to talk about.

Apart from the obvious physical differences, men and women are two completely different species in that we think differently. Men tend to struggle to understand their feelings, and worse to actually talk about them, although you may probably already be aware of this.

A man, instead of just using his heart to understand something complicate things further by also using the gut to process feelings, nothing like doing things the easy way.

The problem is that the gut tends to be listened to more than the heart, which does waste so much time, because instead of responding from the heart we go from a gut feeling, a condition that can respond to situations in every way except the way that you are hoping for.

What I'm trying to say in my meandering way is that just because you can see, understand and accept something it doesn't mean that your guy does.

When he is being slow to catch on it is easy to become annoyed with him, the problem is that if he can't understand why you are annoyed with him you could end up pushing him away.

Blaming your man for being slow to express his feelings will make a man pull away

Try not to get annoyed with your guy because he is being slow to express his feelings for you! Just because he is slow to respond, there is a good chance that he could be attracted to you, it's just that he needs a lot longer than you do to understand his feelings for you.

If you try to push him for a response then you could scare him away. Although we have the amazing ability to hide it well, most men do want to find love, we may come across a wee bit slow at times, but although it's probably not always that apparent, even we realize that life will be a whole lot better if we are in a happy and fulfilling relationship.

Now you should understand that the longer it takes to get some form of commitment from your guy, the more angry, frustrated and confused you're going to become.

If he is unable to respond positively to your feelings for him then it's reasonable to suppose that he has no feelings for you. It's then possible that you might give him an ultimatum.

If you deliver an ultimatum then you had better be prepared to move on, and even if he does respond to your threat what kind of relationship will you have from that point onwards?

If you push him too hard to commit

If you think that you have found the one and you want your relationship to move to the next level you cannot do it alone, this has to be something that you both do together, and you have to do it because you want to do it, because it is the natural next step.

Men will pull away faster than the speed of light if they think that they are being pushed into something that they are not comfortable with, or are not yet ready for. Sometimes you just have to be patient.

Scared of another break-up

Is it possible that the reason that he pulls away is that he has been unlucky in love? It could also be that he has seen far too many people split up, and he doesn't want to pour his heart out to you only to lose you down the road.

If it's the case that your guy has been hurt before, and not found closure from that and possibly ensuing relationships, then he is really going to struggle to create any kind of deep, meaning-ful relationship as he could just be waiting for the point that he breaks up yet again.

It could be the case that he is scared to get to close to you just in case you leave him, and he has to go through all the hurt again. So if he finds himself getting too close to you he could start to pull away rather than risk going through the hurt again.

Earlier on; the importance of communication was mentioned, and it really is so important that that you forgive that it is mentioned again. Unless things have changed, the biggest threat to a marriage or a relationship is a breakdown in communication.

When the communication breaks down then you don't have a relationship, and if a man thinks that he's not in a relationship then he will pull away from you. Properly talking to each other connects you, it forms the bonds that bind you, if you don't talk then you have no connection.

Whilst your guy might be a bit of a Neanderthal when it comes to talking about feelings, there is nothing wrong with sharing your feelings, there is nothing wrong with talking about hopes and dreams.

When you talk you help your relationship grow, you can identify and deal with any problems, you can give yourselves long-term goals for the relationship. When you talk you bring your relationship to life, when you stop it withers away.

Is a lack of communication the reason why men pull away?

So we've dealt with the importance of communication, but there is another part of communication that is just as important as talking, and that's listening to what your partner has to say.

To some degree we all have our own egos and if we have something to say we want to know that people are listening to us.

Men like to be listened to, women like to be listened to, and so if your man thinks that he's not being listened to then he could pull away with his pride all hurt and wounded so that he can have a good sulk.

Regardless of who's saying it, if one of you have something to say then the other should want to listen, because what is important to you should be important to them. But have you ever noticed just how difficult it is to actively listen?

If you're interested in what's being said then you are more likely to listen. If you're not that interested then your face will assume a blank stare (ah body language, don't you just love it and the neat way that it reveals what you are thinking), you probably won't take much notice, but you will make vague non-committal grunts just to give the impression that you are listening.

The worst thing is when you are arguing, because instead of listening to what your partner is saying, you are more likely to be considering the best way to respond.

Regardless of how interesting or not you find the subject make sure that you give your full attention, ask questions, clarify points.

When you actively listen to someone, apart from giving them the same courtesy that you would expect from them, you are showing that you care, you are showing that what matters to them is also important to you, and if your guy knows that you genuinely care about what he thinks then he is going to feel a lot closer to you.

At some point you are going to argue. There is nothing wrong with arguments that clear the air and highlight issues, they help you both deal with problems and to move your relationship forward.

For whatever reason you are having an argument, instead of just confining yourself to the problem at hand you start to bring up every issue and past misdeed that he has committed, needless to say, this is not a healthy way to argue.

Men will pull away from someone who nags, someone who can't leave the past in the past, this sounds a bit harsh, but men will pull away from a drama queen.

Lashing out when he makes mistakes

No one is perfect, everyone makes mistakes, but you have to learn from your mistakes and move on.

Depending on what has happened it doesn't mean that you have to forgive him, but if you want your relationship to survive you have to leave the past in the past, and until you can do that and move your life forward, you will be stuck in limbo.

Lashing out for reasoning differently

You need to accept the fact that you think differently to your man. It's a fact of life that you will have far too many times when you view situations differently to your man, and no matter how many subtle hints you drop he still seems lost.

After a while it can be only too easy to lash out in anger and try to punish him for not understanding you. Whilst your frustration can be justified, the end result is that your man could pull away, because no one likes getting grief for no apparent (to them) reason at all.

If you want to be able to move things forward then as difficult as it may be, you have to learn to understand your man.

Trying to change him

You have to be able to accept him, warts and all for who he is, because that is the guy that you fell in love with. You have to be able to resist any urges to change him to some kind of fantasy ideal.

You may succeed in changing him into someone unlike the man you fell in love with, or worse, what happens if he won't cooperate, what happens if he wants to remain the man you fell in love with?

On the whole men will always pull away from someone who is trying to warp who they are. Be happy with the man you fell in love with, there must be a reason that (even with his faults) that you love him.

Losing his freedom

Men will pull away if they feel that their freedom is under threat so you need to ensure that you both have the opportunity to follow your own lives.

Whilst you won't be able to spend the same amount of time on your hobbies and interests, meeting friends and what have you,

you both still need to do it as that was what made you, you (Hope that makes sense).

Having his own personal space will make him realize that he will not lose who he is, and that he can still be who he is. If he is less likely to fear the loss of his freedom then he is much less likely to need to go off to find himself.

There will be jerks (that's me being very polite) and no matter how much time you invest in the relationship you will never make it work. If you have the misfortune to be stuck with a jerk then please move on and find someone you can be happy with.

If he feels not appreciated

Men will pull away if they feel that they are not appreciated or not listened to, we are such sensitive souls. So let him know that you love him. Let him know that you love him for the unique individual that he is.

Let him know that you are interested in who he is and in his thoughts, feelings, hopes and dreams.

You need to understand that when a man falls in love it can make him feel vulnerable, which for a male psyche could be a very scary thing, so he pulls back, not because he doesn't love you, but because he fears losing himself.

If he is taken out of his comfort zone

Why do men pull away? Thinking on it, it could be that we're just big kids. When we are in an environment that we understand such as out with friends, or maybe playing with computer games, then we are at one with the world.

The problem begins when we are taken out of our comfort zone into a world that is, alien to us, a world where we have to confront our feelings, a world where the happy carefree days of being single have no place, because now instead of only looking after our own wants and needs we have to share, share our lives, our hopes and our dreams.

We know that this new way of living can be good, we realize that it can makes us happy, but for whatever weird, irritating, frustrating reason it can be very difficult to embrace the life that we want, and that we need.

Men pull away for reasons that might not even be known to them, be patient with him, try to understand him, don't try to enclose him, and make him feel wanted and appreciated.

HOW TO DISTINGUISH BETWEEN A MAN WHO'S INTERESTED IN SEX VS. INTERESTED IN YOU

Do Men Just Want Sex?
You have just met this great guy and he has taken you on a few dates. You have known each other for a couple weeks and you really like him. This particular evening, you have ended up at your place on your cozy couch, watching a movie.

The movie has ended, and all of a sudden things have gotten steamy. He is making moves and you feel that he wants to go all of the way.

All of a sudden, all kind of questions enter your mind: Do I really want this? Is this too soon? Is he going to like me the next day? Does he just want sex from me? How do I know if he really likes me? Do I really want to have sex? Am I really enjoying this? What is he really thinking? Do men just want sex? What should I do?

Have you ever had any of these thoughts? If you are like most women, you probably have. Well, want an honest guy's perspective? Want to know what goes through the guy's mind in this situation? Read on!

Before we start, let's clear up something right off. Do men just want sex? No. But many women complain that guys only want sex. And unfortunately, some guys feel bad about this and decide to suppress their sexual drive, when, in fact, there should be nothing wrong with guys wanting to have sex.

It is completely normal and the truth is, yes, most guys do want to have sex. After all, women, you would not want to get a guy who is not sexually interested in you, right?

So, if that is the truth, how do you know if you are having sex too soon, if he actually likes you, if he is going to call you the next day, and what he's really thinking about?

As a disclaimer, I would like to say that the following advice is mainly for those that choose to have sex before marriage. Ultimately, the advice is always to follow your heart.

If in your heart you believe that waiting to be married before having sex is the right thing for you, then the easy answer for you is just to wait.

Don't let anyone tell you otherwise just because it may seem as if everyone else is quick to jump into bed or because the media is so explicit about sex.

But for those of you who are struggling with the decision about when is the right time to have sex, keep reading.

Believe it or not, we guys are very simple creatures. The truth is that we often don't think much before we do something, especially in situations where all of our blood is flowing down south, away from the brain.

So, now that we've covered what is going on in a guy's mind in the heat of the moment, let's help you generally understand men, because the more you understand us, the better decisions you will make for yourself.

Remember that ultimately all that we want is to make you happy. But it's very hard, if not impossible, to respect your wants and wishes, if you don't express them or respect them yourself.

Just because a man wants to have sex with you and is physically attracted to you, does not necessarily mean that he also feels an emotional, mental, and/or spiritual attraction as well.

Healthy chemistry and attraction between men and women often develop differently. Men usually get attracted to women first physically and only after that, mentally and emotionally.

Women, on the other hand, usually first develop a mental or emotional attraction, and only after that does the physical part kick in. But I should also add that it's not always the case for both male and female but most times, generally speaking; that's how it breaks down to.

So, this explains why women can easily misinterpret men's advances of wanting to have sex as meaning that he must also care for her.

Since, intuitively, the woman would generally want sex only if she felt that she really cared for the guy, she is now going to assume the same is true for the guy, in reverse.

So, before having sex, make sure you are not mistakenly setting yourself up to be hurt. Don't assume that because he is physically attracted to you, he also really cares for you.

The second piece of advice explains why waiting to have sex later on can be a win-win situation. Women often make another mistake in thinking that if you don't have sex with a man, his interest in you will drop.

This is simply not true. Although, it is true that men do want to have sex, it is also true that waiting to have sex at a later time can actually increase the passion in your relationship and work to your benefit.

Many women have either heard stories of men leaving their friends-or have experienced this themselves-for reasons of not having had any sex. This automatic association simply is not true.

While there are many men that are looking for just sex, and while it is of course true that if you did date one of these men they would probably leave you because you did not have sex with them, the men that care for you will not leave you for that reason.

And if you were looking for a more serious relationship, you would just be glad that those who were looking for sex did actually leave. If a man really likes you for who you are and cares about you, as you are dating he would not leave you because of no sex.

Some of you may already doubt what is been said, but let's explain further. Over the past ten years, I have seen, experienced, and come in contact with an increasing number of very nice and caring guys who want to make a relationship work just as much as women do.

The truth is that men today also yearn for a satisfying, loving, and happy relationship. While there are also many jerks that often give men a bad name, I have almost daily come in contact with many really nice guys who truly want to make relationships work.

Although these men, if they did date you and liked you, would probably want to have sex with you, they would not leave you just because you wanted to wait while getting to know each other.

In fact, the more they get to like and know you, the more they would probably want to make the occasion special as well. Realize that for a guy to wait to have sex actually helps him search out how much he would want to be intimate with you. This gives the passion in your relationship a chance to grow even more.

There is wisdom in waiting. As you wait to have sex with him, he will have the opportunity to first find out whether he really likes and cares about you.

If you are able to make your dating experiences positive without sex, this delayed gratification will also help him through those tough times in your relationship when you are not seeing eye-to-eye.

The more he experiences being successful in making you happy while you are dating, the more he will have the confidence in himself when times get tough and you are not always as happy with him as in the beginning.

Realize that waiting to have sex for the time when you feel you are ready can help increase the passion in your relationship and assist your guy to become the best man he can be. As long as he feels hope and he has succeeded in making you happy, there is no threat in saying no to his advances.

So, if in the heat of the moment you feel that you are not ready, this is what you can safely say:

"Hey, I really like you and this feels so good, but I am not ready to go further yet. I just like to go slow."

By saying this, you have communicated that you want him to wait, yet you have also done it in a way that also tells him that he has made you happy. In fact, you've given him the courage to continue to pursue you. Should he disregard your wishes, repeat the phrase and be firm.

It is important that you communicate your wants in a way that does not make him wrong for wanting sex, but at the same time makes it clear to him that you expect him to respect you as well.

The more mature you are and the better you know yourself, the easier it is for you to know the right time for you.

How Do I Find a Guy Who Is Not Just Interested In Sex?
That is a very difficult question. Ultimately all men want sex, any man that says otherwise is a liar.

But I presume you mean a man that wants a long term relationship, rather than just a few months of sex or a one night stand. I will explain the things to watch out for.

Flashy guys

You know the ones with a BMW sports car (should be screaming out £20,000 in debt), poser, God's gift to women and has a gift when it comes to chatting up women. The women just converge on these guys and his friends.

Well you know for a fact that if this guy is surrounded by women, he has got no shortage of interested women. Therefore you can be a bit more intelligent than the average woman and realize this guy is just going to move from one woman to the next.

Not the type of guy you want a long term relationship with. Unless you fancy being a single mother, bankrupt because of his flashy cars and friends with the dozens of other single mothers he has deceived.

A lot of women tend to go for the wrong type of men. They always go for men that have girlfriends or are married. That's a problem. To go out with you, they are usually the unfaithful type that are only interested in sex.

Usually they will use you as a bit on the side for a few months without telling their girlfriend or wife. At best they will dump their girlfriend or wife for you, the problem is when the next best woman comes along, you are the one getting dumped.

Unfaithful men cannot be reformed (in most cases) so don't bother with them!

So how do you find the faithful men that are not just interested in sex. Well you make friends with as many men as possible. Just keep them as friends until you know for certain.

Gradually over time they will leak whether they are just interested in sex or whether they want a long term relationship. There are no hard and fast rule to this, most guys can be extreamly patient just to have there with you.

Believe me there are men out there that want long term relationships, but most won't openly admit it. Usually the older a man gets the more mature he gets and the more likely he will be looking for a long term relationship.

You can also pick out from their friends what type of bloke a man is. Usually a friend will say something like "Steven hasn't had any sex for years, poor guy" Jokingly.

You can immediately derive from this sentence that the guy saying he thinks he can get sex whenever he wants and Steven has not had any sex for a while. So to you, Steven should immediately show potential.

The thing here is; if he has gone years without sex, waiting another few months while he is going out with you is not going to make much difference to him. If it does make a difference having to wait for sex then he obviously doesn't value your relationship, so get rid of him.

WHY MEN WITH SWAGGER ARE MORE ATTRACTIVE TO WOMEN – AND HOW TO WEAN YOURSELF OFF OF THEIR ADDICTIVE QUALITIES

Many women would dump their nice and gentlemanly men for men with swagger. Some women are even drawn only to this type of personality.

This fact is pretty bewildering, as a woman is innately predisposed to choose a man who can provide her a sense of security and who she can spend the rest of her life with.

The Psychology of Attraction may provide some useful answers to this interesting development.

People want to be with someone who is different, someone who is the complete opposite of themselves.

Nice women are attracted to men who live with an intoxicating lifestyle because they also want to be a part of that edgier world. That is why a bookworm often gets attracted to a person who rides a Harley.

Nice men also tend to fall for strong-willed women. Such a situation creates a sense of excitement that you cannot feel if you are going out with the same-personality type as yours.

Romance novels influence women like no other. After reading tons of Harlequin romance, there is a huge chance that you would want a man who has a signature swagger and stride with overflowing bravado.

And why not? In most novels, these indifferent, powerful, bold, and mysterious men often become the dreamy, faithful, and loving partner that every woman dreams of.

Women love men who are risk-takers because, most often than not, risk-taking men are successful. They bring home the bacon and are therefore, good providers.

According to anthropologists who are studying the evolutionary traits of people, men who are successful and risk takers often get most of the mating opportunities. Women's primal instincts prefer men who have the best fighting skills, adventurous, and passionate.

Naturally occurring; men with swagger are considered to have a dark triad of personality traits, which include three dominant traits: narcissism, psychopathic, and Machiavelli.

Based on these traits, men with swagger exhibit common behavior like indifference, egotism, cynicism, manipulative and deceptive behavior, callousness, selfishness, thrill-seeking impulsiveness, lack of empathy, and superficial charms.

The James Bond character is one example of an alpha male with dark triad traits. These traits are also often the character traits of male protagonists in romance novels.

According to research, men with dark triad personality traits know how to manipulate women, making them dangerous and interestingly, appealing to most women. Many psychologists believe that men with swagger can activate the mother's instincts, and as a result, women feel compassion and want to take care of these men with the hope of changing their unappealing attitude (if there's any) for the better.

Despite all these seemingly negative traits, women still fall for guys like this

How to wean yourself off men with swagger addictive qualities

A man who has some swag may come across as arrogant, but if he has the looks, attitude and everything else to pull it off, he becomes a heart-throb.

Every woman innately wants a man who can handle himself in situations, and who has the confidence and ability to be a success, because this is the kind of man who can provide a stable future.

Confident men are looked up to which gives them status and power, and is sexy. It's exactly the same the other way round if you think about it. Men are attracted to confident women.

If you are seeing one of these guys and he has lost interest in you, it is probably because you were easy to manipulate, and once his quest has been achieved and you have been devoured he's ready to move on to the next.

The thing is, while confidence and power are certainly attractive qualities to begin with, they are not enough to form a man who can fill all of a woman's needs. A woman naturally seeks security on a mental and emotional level too.

Swagger men are seriously lacking in this area which is why you will never, ever be one hundred per cent fulfilled with him. If you want to find true happiness then you need a fully-rounded man. Swagger men are not fully developed men. Fully developed and fully-rounded up man has style not swagger.

Here are how to wean yourself off his addictive qualities:

The thrill factor

• Every swagged men comes with the thrill factor. There's the chase and the challenge, the excitement and risk, the spontaneous high-speed romance swagger men naturally ooze that mysterious quality, it's like you never can get quite close enough to touch them.

They're also experts at seduction and manipulation. They know how to use all of their attractive traits to get exactly what they want out of a woman. He will make you feel amazing for the time that you are in his line of vision, but due to his high-speed tendencies and lack of focus, he won't stick around for long.

Suddenly you're the one chasing him! The best thing for you is to get it into your head that it is the thrill factor that attracts them, as well as you. As soon as you become a sure thing, you're not a challenge anymore.

They don't want predictable, safe, or boring. They want to be on the go. Can you deal with this? Are you willing to constantly be reinventing yourself to fit into the needs of a man who needs the constant thrill of the chase?

Or can you accept that as a long-term plan it would be exhausting, unsatisfying and unrealistic? You want more than this. You deserve more. Re-evaluate your needs and find a man that fits them.

The Emotional Roller Coaster

• Heightened emotions can become dangerously addictive, whether they are good or bad, you will get to a point where even the lows feel good because they are so intense that nothing compares.

Some women feed off feelings of intense anger, jealousy and insecurity. Why? Well it's certainly not boring! Once you have become accustomed to feeling a constant imbalance of intense emotions to each extreme, any ordinary feeling is dull and doesn't have quite the same kick.

Women like this mistake these emotions for 'love'. The most important thing to know is that it is not exactly healthy to be feeling so high and then so low with such intense frequency.

Think about the effect it could be having on all of your other relationships, which should be just as important. Is it affecting your work life? Your productivity at home? Your social scene?

Are these not just as important as being in a relationship? You have to understand that a happy and healthy life is about finding a good balance. If your relationship is taking up so much of your energy, then it is only your own life that is being robbed, not his.

Choose Compatibility Over Chemistry

• Chemistry can grow as you get to know someone better. However, it's unlikely that you'll actually become more compatible with someone over time. Swagger men usually provide a GLIMPSE of something that you want and then snatch it away. Real compatibility i.e. wanting the same things as someone else doesn't go. It simply is.

Get Excited About Your Own Life

• When women complain of always attracted to swagger men, one thing they mention is that they "get bored" with regular men so swagger men seem so attractive and different. Prevent this by getting passionate about creating an awesome life of your own.

When you're passionately interested in your own life, the swagger men will represent a hazard rather than a creative way to stave off boredom. Stop writing off stable men as boring.

Take a Wait and See Approach

• Don't commit, jump into anything, or declare any guy "The One" in the first few months of being together. Swagger men will either be totally glib about commitment and refuse to take it seriously or they'll push for it right away to tie you down and obligate you to stick around.

Obviously, neither is a recipe for success. Time is your ally. You'll learn everything you need to know if you sit back and pay attention without doing anything permanent.

HOW WHAT YOU SHOULD BE LOOKING FOR IN A PARTNER IS VERY DIFFERENT FROM WHAT YOU HAVE BEEN LOOKING FOR IN A PARTNER

Are you with someone, married, or in committed relationships? Are you tired of being the odd one out, tired of being alone? Do you think that you are missing out on something, do you think that there is more to life than what you have?

Are you ready to dive into the first chance of a relationship that you get, or will you look for the right person? Do you know if you are ready for a serious relationship?

When you go into a relationship you have to give up a lot. When you are single, you can pretty much do what you want. When you are single, all of your decisions revolve around what is best for you. Are you ready to give all of that up?

Do you have you own life, your own friends, your own hobbies and interests. The chances are that you do, which is great, because it makes you a more interesting person. How will you manage this life when you are in a relationship?

Is your life so busy that you will struggle to find time for a relationship? Are you ready to compromise on what you do so that you can spend time with your partner?

No-one can expect you to give up your friends and interests, but if you are ready for a serious relationship then they have to take second place to your partner.

Are you ready to commit, and forsake all others? It's a massive step committing to one person, building a relationship into which you pour your energy. How do you view commitment, does it scare you?

You know if you are ready for a serious relationship if you can understand the happiness and fulfillment to be found in a committed, intimate relationship.

Do you have realistic expectations of your serious relationship, or have you been influenced by what you see in the movies, see on the T.V, or read in books. Stories portray an ideal world and not reality.

Can you find someone to love for who they are, and not what you want them to be. Can you work to make your relationship the very best that it can be given your life, location, and circumstances, and not try to make it into something that it is not?

Are you comfortable with who you are? Or is it a case that you do not believe that anyone could be interested in you, so you try to come across as someone you are not? In order to be ready for a serious relationship you have to be happy with who you are, and comfortable with yourself.

If you are not, how can you expect anyone else to be? There are things that you can change through study, or going to the gym, but your core person cannot be changed so be happy and confident with yourself.

If you try to be someone you are not, then if someone falls for that person you will have a difficult time in maintaining your character. Don't start your relationship with a lie, be yourself.

Have you had some bad experiences in previous relationships, and have you managed to achieve closure on those experiences?

If you have not managed closure, then you will be dragging your baggage from relationship to relationship, and it will keep getting heavier, because until you can deal with your issues and leave them in the past, then you will not be able to move forward.

If you are ready for a serious relationship then you can understand that your new relationship is a blank canvas. Whatever has happened in previous relationships, whether good or bad has nothing to do with this one.

You and your new partner are building something new together, and to make that happen you both need to work together and build to the future, and not let your relationship be affected by what has happened in the past.

How to know if you are ready for a serious relationship

If you are just looking for a security blanket, someone to make you feel better about yourself, then you are most certainly not ready. You are ready for a serious relationship if you want to find someone who you can share your life with.

You are ready for a serious relationship if you are prepared to commit to one, if you are prepared to devote the time and energy that it will take you.

You know that you are ready for a serious relationship if you are not heading for the hills as soon as the word commitment is mentioned.

And finally, you know that you are ready for a serious relationship if you realize that a life with someone special at your side is a life worth living.

What to Look For in a Partner

Relationships are very important. They help us to learn more about ourselves and about people of the same or different nationalities, races, tribes, and genders. It will be very difficult and even impossible for courtship or marriage to take place without a relationship between one person and another.

For love relationship to take place and flourish; there are many things that must be incorporated in a relationship that is intended to become a love relationship. Later parts of this work give the stages that love relationship should follow.

No two relationships are exactly alike or develop in just the same way; however, healthy relationships have some things in common. First, each partner in a healthy relationship must have a positive self-image. Once you feel strong and sure of yourself, you are in better position to know what to look for in a partner.

Second, you should be aware; always that love develops in stages. Love cannot be rushed. Once you find an appropriate partner, do not give in to the temptation to try "Hurry things along" by skipping early phases of development. These early times provide the foundation of a strong relationship later on. Be patient.

Many relationships and marriages got broken up because the partners were not patient during the beginning stages of their relationships. They did not take time to study each other comprehensively.

Their lack of patience made them not to know much of the likes and dislikes of one another or characters that would be ignored, tolerated or not tolerated. When conflicts arose, they were unable to be resolved amicably thereby leading to the severance of the relationships and divorce. In searching for a partner, it is good to look for qualities that can help you establish a lasting relationship and marriage.

In thinking about a person who interests you, you should make sure that the person has time and energy available for love. Such people:

- Are not involved in other love relationships.

- Have not just recently broken up with someone else.

- Are open to be in a relationship with you.

- Are free of chemical or psychological addictions (people with addictions to alcohol or other drugs, people who gamble, or with eating disorders cannot function well in love relationships).

- Have time to devote to a relationship.

• Have high self-esteem

• Are close to you geographically - they live in your city or state.

In addition, the person must be compatible with you in terms of social values and beliefs.

To evaluate these factors, see if you can honestly answer yes to the following questions:

• Does the person have several close friends? A person who has learned to keep and enjoy close relationships can put this talent to work in a love relationship.

• If the relationship folded, would you still want that person as a friend? Without friendship, the relationship may crumble during times of conflict.

• Are you happy with the way the person treats other people? Watch how the person deals with school employees, waitresses, maids, sales clerks, telephone operators, and close friends.

If you would not want to be on the receiving end of that behavior, do not get involved. You may be an exception during courtships, but you will not be later on.

You can be friends with people who lack these qualities, but beware of deeper relationships until these problems are resolved. Also, be sure that you are available for a relationship because if you are too busy to be close to your partner in a relationship, it will lack the time and energy it needs to grow.

THE DOWNSIDE IN LOOKING FOR
A MAN WHO HAS EVERYTHING
IN COMMON WITH YOU

Before going into details about the downside in looking for a man who has everything in common with you I would like to you to keep one thing in mind.

If you want to date a smart, strong, successful man, his greatest concern isn't necessarily whether you have a Masters' degree or Phd, speaks more than three languages, or have a summer home in the Hamptons. It's how he feels around you, how happy he is around you.

Most men ultimately gravitate toward women who make them feel sexy, funny and trusted. But don't get it wrong that doesn't mean men are not attracted to the female version of themselves in terms of intellectual, liberal, passionate, opinionated; it wouldn't just WORK, that's all.

So do intellectual or creative men like intellectual or creative women? No doubt such a man would love his woman to be creative and intelligent too but the problem isn't whether such men will like you or understand you.

The problem is whether your weaknesses will exacerbate each other.

Are you both highly emotional to certain situations? Are you both dreamers? Are you sometimes depressed or even bipolar? Do you run from anything that seems stable because it seems boring?

Do either of you have any practical skills? Will you ever be able to afford to raise children? Because you may be the best of friends, have amazing chemistry, and really "get" each other, but if both of you have the same flaws, the relationship may be untenable.

This is what I mean by compatibility. Understand that having same interests has nothing to do with compatability. Compatibility is about respect.

For example If your man love music, and you don't, you two can be perfectly happy together as long as you don't judge your partner for not loving music or your partner is trying to stop you from loving your music.

The point is So don't worry about whether you're dating someone who is not of the same interest has you or have the same dream or passion as you.

Worry about whether your relationship is easy and whether you're built for the long haul. Your common interests may draw you together but they will not keep you together.

Having the same interests isn't that important when it comes to compatibility. In fact, it's possible to have great chemistry with someone who has almost nothing in common with you!

What matters most is that both parties are respectful and accepting of each other's beliefs and preferences. In many relationships, people tend to fall into the trap of obsessing over the things they don't have in common with their partner, or even worse, they try to change their partner.

But here's the thing: Being in a relationship does not give anyone the right to mold their partner into the person they want them to be. Unless it's that person's choice or they're willing to change, compromising their interests will only lead to more stress and frustration.

So instead of sticking to this ridiculous myth that shared interests are required to make relationships work, remember that it's more important to be open-minded and just embrace what makes you and your partner so different

Here are some of the Downside In Looking For a Man Who

Has Everything In Common With You.

The conversations would get boring after a while:
• While it's true that common interests usually draw people together and bond them over time, sharing the same interests can lead to some pretty dull and lifeless conversations.

It's especially bad if you find that you and your partner share the same opinions and flaws, because the relationship will probably fizzle out more quickly. Because it would everyday routine thing talking about same thing all the time things both of you already know about.

You wouldn't want to try new things:
• Think about it. If you and your partner have the same interests, you'll probably grow comfortable and stick to the same routine, day in and day out. Unfortunately, this leaves no opportunity for you to explore new things and spice things up a bit, you wouldn't want to get out of your comfort zone because you would feel there is nothing to exploit.

Less adventurous:
• And speaking of comfort zones, since you're so content with doing the same things over and over again, you probably don't even think about the fact that your relationship lacks excitement and adventure.

Being adventurous gives you and your partner the chance to explore new interests together! And when your relationship lacks excitement and adventure it brings it back to the first problem it would become boring.

Again, sticking to the same hobbies, having the same conversations and agreeing on everything is a surefire way to get bored pretty fast. But this is less likely to happen with someone who encourages you to try something new and see things a little differently.

Most time it feels like you are dating yourself:

• Do you remember when Justin Timberlake soulfully sings about it, it's hard to believe that dating a mirrored version of yourself is not the best thing in the world. But hear me out:

Dating a carbon copy of yourself can eventually get really boring, because nothing would excite you you would just be there for example if you are a workaholic or worry too much about certain situation of things that happen and your man too is same their wont be that feeling that you have someone who can actually console you not to worry anymore with his sweet words but if you are dating someone opposite he would know how to pamper and make you feel you are not alone in the situation.

You wont feel challenged:
• It can be so exciting to be with someone who has opinions that mostly differ from yours, because then, it challenges you to reconsider your own views and start interesting discussions.

This doesn't mean that you and your partner should get into a full-blown fight over issues that you don't agree on. Rather, you can respectfully agree to disagree and accept these differences.

You would probably get tired of the relationship on a long run:
• At first, it may feel like a dream. You're so happy that you've found this person and they're so similar to you that they feel like an extension of yourself. But in time, that feeling often fades.

If you're not with someone who challenges you to be a little different, to think outside the box, or to consider new perspectives, then things are going to fizzle out fast because every one loves to be pampered one way or the order.

So, always remember that Opposites attract. It helps to have some common interests, something about which both halves of a couple can enjoy together. But the differences are what keeps a relationship interesting, and the individuals from going mad.

Having one's own interests means having something to pursue alone and having alone-time is important. It also allows the individuals to have an "identity" or "role" within the relationship, enhancing the trust, reliance and enjoyment of each other's company.

WHY MEN ARE HEAD-CENTERED
MORE THAN HEART-CENTERED

There is hopefully a lot of honesty and authenticity in any meaningful relationship, but there does seem to be selective omissions of information that occur in every marriage.

Either intentionally (not wanting to rock the boat) or unintentionally (not understanding the importance of this information to one's spouse), men don't always say what they feel.

In fairness, we guys do have difficulty verbalizing our emotions, reasons women see us as being head-centered and not heart centered and this is due to a socialization issue we have as a society, that devalues this strength, painting it as a weakness in boys.

While adults in therapy do have the ability to make significant gains in openness, communication and self insight, not every man has had this experience, and thus will need some help.

Women can take an active role in modeling verbalization of affection, and make efforts to strongly reinforce and acknowledge the efforts that are made.

While most us are not perfect, if women were to look, there are countless examples of attempts their husband's have made to please them (even as simple as agreeing to watch one of "her shows" or participate in activities she loves), it just may not be the verbalization she hoped for.

Rewarding a behavior will naturally increase it, and there are lots of ways to show your husband he's appreciated. Pointing out specifically, the things you appreciate will provide encouragement to continue down this path. In this case, omission may not be intentional, and just needs encouragement and training.

Typically, with us, we tend to minimize importance of our female friends to our spouses or omit altogether. Through these platonic relationships, we can derive positive insight into the opposite gender that is invaluable.

The importance of these friendships is often minimized to our wives, due to what we perceive will be a jealous and aggressive response.

Women can model openness to social interactions including making efforts to engage their husband's friends, while also reinforcing the strength of their own relationship with their husband, and talking about appropriate boundaries she feels comfortable with.

Jealousy smells like insecurity and this can create a self-fulfilling prophecy. The space you create will determine the safety your partner feels to disclose.

We often minimize or altogether omit their true feelings about sex, and what excites us. Women who pass judgment on what turns her man on, or worse, puts them in a position of shame, is sure to open the door for dishonesty or withdrawal.

Minimizing the power of the sex drive is foolish. If the discussion of sex is taboo, then it opens in other areas like pornography, or possibly emotional affairs online or at work. Don't be scared to talk about sex.

We often minimize or are reluctant to talk about our financial concerns. This happens for a number of reasons, but a common thing is men being scared to disappoint, or a fear they will be seen as someone who does not provide.

So much of a man's self-esteem is derived from his earning power, and this is on display all the time with every interaction that is had with other couples, or if there are kids, with other families.

Reinforcing that you are a team, and that you will survive anything together, can provide the safety for us to open up about our fears, and sources of anger and hurt. This openness can lead to collaborative decision-making, and reduce unnecessary stress.

While we may appear withdrawn in these areas, it is something wives can fix. Negative criticism or strong responses do not lead to the results people hope for. Meeting a person where they are, modeling what you want to see, and reinforcing safety is always the best path.

KNOWING WHAT IS "GOOD ENOUGH" IN A MAN AND WHEN IT'S A REASONABLE COMPROMISE

Compromise seems to be a dirty word these days. Women deserve the best! They should never settle! It has to be Mr. Good, not Mr. Good Enough. But does "good enough" mean settling? Everyone has flaws; why should one expect Mr. Good not to have a few flaws too? Surely that just makes him human?

Women shouldn't be holding out for "Mr. Good" but should hook up with "Mr. Good Enough". Why waste your life on useless dates and meaningless flings, always thinking that your prince is around the corner, when you can settle for someone who ticks most of the "boxes" and isn't too bad?

There are so many really wonderful men out there, men who want commitment, who want to be married, who are attractive and smart and interesting. They may not be movie-star attractive, they may be awkward at first, they may not fit your cultural image of who Mr. Good is or who Prince Charming is. But you shouldn't pass them up.

There are two kinds of people in the world: maximizers and satisfiers. Maximizers are not good when it comes to dating and entering relationships (and staying in them!) whereas satisfiers are. Schwartz, social scientist uses a shopping analogy to explain this theory. Two women, one a maximizer and one a satisfier, decide to go shopping for a new jumper.

Both have very clear criteria of what this sweater should look like, how much it should cost and how it should feel (v-neck, not itchy, pink, etc.). The satisfier walks into one or two stores, finds a sweater that meets all of her criteria and buys it.

She's done and is satisfied with her purchase. And how is the maximizer woman doing? Well, she has walked in and out of at least five stores. She found a sweater that matched all her criteria in the first store she went into, but she thought she should check out the store down the street just to be sure... and the store next door.

And maybe one more. Maybe she can find a better one. Maybe she can find a better one on sale. Two hours later she thinks she has found The sweater so she finally makes the decision and buys it.

So who is happier with their sweater? Most people would say, obviously the maximizer; she looked longer, was more discerning and explored more options.

Wrong! In the end the satisfier will always be happier with her purchase as she knows she got the best she wanted; whereas, the maximizer will always wonder if she really did get the absolute best one. A satisfier isn't looking for the absolute best but she does still have high standards.

The difference is that she stops when she has found something that meets those high standards. She doesn't wonder if she can do better if she looks longer.

So what's more important? Holding out for Mr. Right, acting like a maximizer? Or be a satisfier and pick Mr. Good Enough, confident in your decision? And do we even need these labels?

The concept of happily ever after has been taken over by Hollywood and that no "real" relationship can live up to the expectations of those who watch the romantic movies churned out year after year.

Perhaps Mr. Good is Mr. Good Enough and perhaps he's a real man with real flaws and (more importantly) real feelings, which is ultimately what every woman wants.

WHAT HAPPENED TO THE GUYS YOU WERE THE "MOST" ATTRACTED TO

Disaster after dating disaster, you just can't seem to find the right guy. Every guy you've been attracted to up until today has been a complete waste of time, and probably left you feeling extremely hurt and damaged. Worse yet, is the fact that lots of these guys have dumped you, or have stopped calling...and you don't know why.

But that is all about to change, as you will be getting an insight into a man's mind that will show you exactly why you are only attracting the wrong types of guys.

You see, there are certain things that women do which determine which type of man they can have; and clearly, if you are attracting the wrong kind of guy, you are not sending off the signals that would attract the right guy.

Let's look at these 25 tips and see if you can identify with them, because chances are, you're doing more than one of these things which is causing you to attract the wrong type of guy:

#1. You don't draw the boundaries-
If a man wants to get intimate with you, he can. If he wants to disrespect you or make fun of you, he can. If he wants to say he'll call but never does, he can. He walks all over you, because he can, and because you let him. Draw the boundaries, otherwise you'll find that men will do whatever they want to, regardless of how

you feel about it.

#2. You tell them not to like you, because you don't like yourself-

You give off the vibe that you really hate yourself, and that you don't value yourself. You downsize yourself and show your insecurities in your self-sabotaging comments and jokes that you make about yourself when you talk to men. This tells them that you are a low quality woman, and thus they treat you like one.

#3. You jump into bed too early –

You try to snag him by jumping into bed with him, but that only backfires when you realize that he only wanted a one night stand. Never become intimate with a man early on, if he is truly into you, he won't make that a requirement, and will not rush into intimacy with you.

#4. You don't think you can accomplish your goals without a man-

You want a house, and kids, and a stable life...and you sit there telling men how you need to settle down with a guy just to get these things. This comes across as being utterly needy and even creepy at times; and tells him that you're not really willing to give yourself anything on your own, and instead expect a man to give you the life you desire.

#5. You expect commitment instantly -

You just met the guy, and already you are strangling him with commitment talks and expectations. The quickest way to scare a man off is by making him feel as though you are trying to trap him; which talking about commitment does!

If a man wants to commit, he doesn't want to be told to do it; but wants to choose it, which you don't allow him to do when you come on too strong in the beginning.

#6. You're extremely bossy –

You talk about all the things he has to do for you, and get for you, and he thinks you're just a spoiled brat who needs to grow up. He's never going to let you boss him around or tell him what to do, and will probably throw that in your face just to teach you a lesson.

#7. You don't give him space –

A man will become a complete jerk when you deprive him of space and when you deprive him of his "personal" time alone and away from you. Men will literally argue and cause a huge fight just to have a valid reason to leave you, because otherwise, they'd never be able to get some time alone.

#8. You're too touchy –

He says one small thing and it offsets you so much that you start crying, or argue for 3 hours about it, and you just can't drop anything or let anything go. He doesn't want to feel like he's walking on egg shells around you, so instead he will just dump you on the sidelines and find someone who isn't so touchy.

#9. You let him take you for granted –

You give him so much so early on, without him having to earn it or work for it, that he starts to take you for granted. His ego is inflated because he is getting you to do everything for him, without working for it...thus he literally doesn't appreciate you, and you mean nothing to him...because it's just you who is chasing him. He'll treat you like crap as a result.

#10. You let men determine your mood –

Your mood depends entirely on what other men think, and whether or not they are attracted etc... Thus, if you are rejected or if he doesn't call you... you will instantly feel down. Likewise, if he talks to you for a while, or if he says he likes you... your mood elevates.

Men notice this behavior and may play around with you just to get a reaction... which in turn means they are not genuine but instead are entertaining themselves at the cost of your pain.

#11. You're too submissive –

While it's true that men want to be in control; the issue is that when you are too submissive men become control hungry because they become used to the idea of controlling you.

Thus, when you try to gain control, they only become worse and try to control you more, because their comfort zone rests in having control over everything because you started off being submissive and thus conditioned them to only want you when you are submissive.

Therefore, they never let you make decisions, never let you have any say or any control and in turn just abuse you when you try to put your foot down.

#12. You tell men to judge you –

You talk about your problems, your past relationships, your mistakes etc... and then you ask him what he thinks or what his input is; which is like asking him to judge you. He, of course, will judge you, and then will sound like a complete jerk. but, that's your fault, for giving him permission to criticize and judge you so heavily to begin with.

#13. You don't uphold your morals –

You tell a guy that you're a good and clean girl; yet not even 5 minutes later you are acting completely different just to try and win him over, when your first approach doesn't work. Men won't want to commit to women who can't uphold their morals, and would often view these women as being low class, easy takes.

#14. You change everything just to be with a guy –

It's not natural that you're suddenly interested in everything he is, and he notices that it's fake. He knows that you're just pretending and are altering your entire life just to try and show him that you have things in common.

Some guys may take advantage of this in a bad way when they realize it, and may introduce you to bad habits, poor choices, and other things to get what they want.

#15. You don't stand up for yourself –

He'll pick on you or do something that is completely rude, and you don't stand up for yourself, and don't speak up to let him know that it's something you dislike or that it's something unacceptable.

When you don't stand up for yourself, you tell a man that it's alright to continue the behavior, because he doesn't know otherwise, and will probably increase the poor behavior as a result.

#16. You don't respect yourself –

Instead, you expect men to respect you, because that's the only way you can feel good, and the only way you can get respect. but, it starts from within, and a man will never respect a woman who does not respect herself because he doesn't have a reason to.

The only reason a man would do something, is if a woman makes it clear by doing it herself first, at least in this case.

#17. You initiate everything –

Even if he lets you initiate something, it's only because it's easier for him, and it means he can get what he wants with little to no effort. It's every guys dream to have easy girls chasing after them, which is what you appear to be when you initiate everything.

Men who are genuine will always initiate the important things first, such as getting your phone number, taking you on a date, starting a relationship, moving in together etc...

#18. You try to change him –

If you have to change a man, he's clearly not the right guy for you. Put it this way: if he was what you wanted, would you have to change him? While it's true that everyone can improve, nagging a man to change is like saying that who they are right now is not acceptable to you.

If it's not acceptable, why are you chasing him? He won't

change just because you come along and tell him to; instead you'll probably change before he does.

#19. You fail to leave when he doesn't commit –
He dodges the topic of commitment, doesn't want to talk about the future, and runs away from the idea of marriage.

But, you stick around still thinking that it will work out, and that he will do it...but this is when you should leave. You only hurt yourself more when you stay with a man who clearly has no intentions of committing, simply because you hope he will.

#20. You accept the "friendship zone" –
He says that he isn't ready to date again, and tells you that he just wants to stay single. He also tells you that he just wants to be friends instead. Did you ever throw yourself under the bus by accepting that kind of a lie from men.

It's a huge lie and an excuse when men say that they don't want a relationship now, because they are looking, but they just don't want to commit to you.

#21. You want men to fix your life –
You have all kinds of problems and expect men to come in like a valiant knight or magical prince charming and fix everything. Men sense this, and instead of adding to your problems, they rebel and add to your problems.

They don't want to be treated like a doormat that you step on and wipe your feet off on; and they don't want to be part of all the drama that is your own life which you can't even fix on your own.

#22. You use men –
Men get the vibe that you use them, because you might only seem to be interested in their money, in their car, in their connections (business, friends, hobbies etc.), or you might treat them like they are a trophy.

They sense this and retaliate in turn by using you back, which means they may just use you for attention, sex, an ego boost etc.

#23. You don't deliver –

You impress him when you first meet, and he gets this idea that you are this amazing chick, because you told him you were... but when he sees you the next time you are just dull, he sees right through you, and ends up thinking you don't deliver.

But, just because you don't deliver on all the things he wants, that doesn't mean that he still can't use you for something or rather, which he will, and when he's finished he'll dump you... which will be pretty fast.

#24. You expect men to entertain you-

You go out with men because you are bored, or want something to do. You are looking for entertainment, and he sees it, when you constantly ask him to take you places...and don't really seem to be interested in him as a person, but rather seem more interested in what entertains you.

This will make him start to disrespect you and lose interest, which in turn makes him not really care about hurting your feelings, because he thinks you don't care either.

#25. You never agree with men –

You think they are wrong most of the time, and always argue with them. They get sick and tired of being nagged, and in turn start to act out against you, because they can't handle it anymore. If you can't ever agree with a man or find some common ground, it should be obvious that he in turn, won't agree with you and will only take his side and want things his way.

IT'S NOT ABOUT THE QUALITY OF THE PERSON, IT'S ABOUT THE QUALITY OF THE RELATIONSHIP

Relationships can be determined by type, quality and purpose. Different types of relationship can have different qualities and a different purpose. This is what makes all relationships individual and unique to those within the relationship.

What type of relationship that you have with someone depends upon the roles that you are both playing within the relationship. As the roles change, so does the type of relationship.

Husband & wife, father & son, mother & daughter are all different types of relationship. Teacher & pupil, trainer & trainee, therapist & client, coach & coachee are all different types of relationship. Director & manager, manager & worker, employer & employee, employee & customer are all different types of relationship as well.

As we change our roles within a relationship, we change the type of relationship that we are having and how we relate to another person.

A mother & daughter may relate to each other as a parent & child during the early years of their relationship and relate to each other as best friends later in life, even though they remain a mother and a daughter by virtue of their ancestral lineage rather than as their roles in life.

The type of relationship does not determine the quality of the relationship. The Quality of a relationship is determined by the compatibility and the co-operation of the individuals within the relationship, rather than the qualities, attributes and attainments of the individuals themselves.

The compatibility and co-operation of the people within a relationship is determined by the **Law of Attraction** according to how alike people are or how attractive they are to each other.

People who are alike, like each other and relate well. They are compatible and they co-operate with each other. Relationships become strained because as well as 'like attracts like', opposites also attract. Gender opposites attract and relate well, whereas polar opposites repel each other and find each other repulsive.

Miserable people can get on well with miserable people, whereas happy people can't. An arrogant person may be seen by their humble partner as confident. A meek person may be seen by an arrogant partner as weak.

The quality of the relationship is not determined by the quality of the emotional state of being of the individuals within the relationship. Neither is it determined by the type of role that the individuals are adopting, nor is it determined by the purpose of the relationship.

By sharing the highest aspects of who you are with another who has attained those attributes, allows you both to experience and to enjoy the exponential benefits of your development and growth. This is called an Interdevelopmental Relationship and is 'Being Together in Togetherness'.

Projecting Onto Your Partner "Negative" or "Positive" Traits and Behaviors Harms the Relationship

When you deny and repress traits and feelings that exist within you, and project them onto your partner, you're liable to harm your relationship. The following are ways that most ladies this in their relationships:

• You identify these traits, feelings, needs and fears in your man.

• You repeatedly accuse him for having traits, feelings, needs and fears that you deny in yourself (being hot tempered; aggressive; arrogant; domineering, etc.). You are certain that you are not stingy, for example, but always argue with your partner about spending money.

• At times you blame him for causing you to become aggressive, dominating, insensitive, etc. ("It's because of you that I...").

• You get angry with yourself for having such a partner.

• You constantly focus on what you don't like in your partner.

• You believe that if your partner changes (if he stops being hot tempered; arrogant; dominating; stingy, needy, fearful, etc.) you'll then have a wonderful relationship.

Usually, when you think in terms of "if only he will change - then", you don't consider, even for a moment, that there might be something within you that needs change. You ask your partner to change; you demand it; you manipulate him to change; sometimes you even threaten ("If you don't..., then...").

When you continually accuse your partner for having traits, emotions, needs and fears that you deny within yourself, get angry with him/her and demand that changes, he/she is liable to react with anger of his/her own and accuse you in a similar way.

As a result, you're liable to find yourself in a mix of frustration, arguments, misunderstandings and mutual recriminations, thus sabotaging your relationship. You fight, become alienated and maybe even leave your partner or are being left.

Projecting harms your relationships

As long as you're not aware of your repressions, denials and projections, you will continue having arguments and conflicts with your partner. If your relationship ends and you begin a new one, sooner or later you will realize that the new relationship is just like the previous one.

• In the beginning of a relationship, you don't see in your new man the traits that "bothered" you in your previous ones.

• Sooner or later, you "discover" that your new man has the same traits that bothered you in our previous ones.

• You get into the same fights and arguments that you had with previous partners.

• You behave the same way you did with your previous partners: you accuse; try to change him; you end the relationship - or your partner does.

Projection of "positive" traits is also harmful to the relationship

When you think about projection, you usually think of "negative" traits. Sometimes, however, you also repress and deny in yourself traits, qualities and emotions which, deep inside you, you see as "positive" (such as: passion, sensitivity, creativity, playfulness, assertiveness, and gentleness).

If during your childhood you've unconsciously internalized that these traits, qualities and emotions are liable to embarrass you, invite criticism, and even prevent you from being loved, you repress and deny them.

As much as you repress and deny them within you, you also wish, at some deep unconscious level, that you had these traits, qualities and emotions. But since you think that you don't, you believe your guy does because:

• Deep inside yourself you perceive these traits, qualities and emotions as "positive". That's why, if you identify them in your man, it means that your man is "ideal".

• You feel "privileged" to go out with somebody "ideal" like him.

• You believe that if your partner has these traits, he/she "completes" you.

But as much as projection of "negative" traits and emotions

harms your relationships, so does projection of "positive" ones.

With time, when you realize that your man doesn't have these traits and qualities, you become bitter, disappointed and angry at him. You also become angry for having deceived yourself. You then begin to focus on the traits that you don't like in your partner.

Regardless of whether you project onto your partners "negative" or "positive" traits, qualities and emotions, as long as you're not aware of it, you will keep doing so. When your relationships continue to collapse one after the other, you are prone to believe and generalize that "all men are the same".

THE DANGER IN LOOKING FOR THE
MALE VERSION OF YOURSELF

You think you know your type. In fact, you are sure of it. You have dated them, perhaps even married them - more than once on both counts. So, if you know your type so well, why are you still looking for Mr. Right?

Get over your type and open your mind, your feelings, and your experiences to seeing who may be right for you. If knowing your type were working so well, you would not be looking. With that harsh realty acknowledged and accepted, are you ready to move on?

Of course, there is the other side of the coin. He's not my type. As well as you think you know your type, you also think you know who is not your type. This is as a big problem in my opinion as knowing who your type is.'

Let me share this with you. If most women had continued to judge potential dates by types, they would not now be married to amazing men and someone who is so perfect for them. When you learn about what it felt like to be with men - it will different, from what you think your type is.

You have to go out of your own way and just trust in the process of knowing the qualities, characteristics, attributes, personality, and way of being together. This will take time and reflection.

You have to stop looking for the version of yourself in men, and begin to open yourself to possibilities. Chemistry grows over time and is based on many factors. Yet, so many women dismiss potential men because they don't "feel" it right away.

If you are basing a lifetime of happiness on whether or not

your heart jolts at first sight, you are selling yourself short and missing out on many opportunities.

Give a man and yourself a chance to interact, talk, and know him before you decide there is no chemistry. The other thing to keep in mind is that we often gravitate to what we know and feels comfortable to us on a subconscious level. Yet, if that were working so well, you would not be single and looking.

It takes courage to try something new and break out of your comfort zone. People, who do, often tell me how happy they are. There is a whole world waiting for you that you don't even know exists and that includes amazing relationships with men. How will you know unless you give it a try?

Sounds easy. Yet if it were, we'd all be with our perfect partners. Divorce would be non-existent. Online dating sites and agencies would not exist and there would be far less singles.

You must look into other people as well as at them. Look into their good, their gifts, and see them. Give yourself and the people you meet this gift and watch the quality of your relationships improve.

Then watch the quality of the men you meet improve. Love is not easy, yet it is glorious when you find it. Open yourself to the possibility of love in people and places you might not expect. Mr. Right is waiting for you.

Mr Right Now - How To Attract A Man That Matches Who You Are, Right Now

#1. List what you bring to the relationship
#2 List what you enjoy doing
#3 List what you value having

Because who we are changes and evolves, so do our needs. As the items on your list change, the person you attract will change; because you have changed. The man who is right for you at this moment, may not be the man who is right for you down the line.

Be open to experiencing happiness fully, right now, so you can focus on the present, and not be distracted by what the future may hold for you.

Be open to being with the man who fits who you are now. Eventually, you will focus on attracting the person who fits with the life you want in the future.

Be true to your nature, right now. Get all the stuff out of the way that you want to experience, and be able to say, "been there, done that." If, right now, you enjoy running the streets at night, drinking with your friends, going to night clubs, you want to know how to attract a man who fits with that lifestyle.

That's what will make you happy, right now. Sometimes, you need to have your current experience to learn about yourself, learn what you really like or to just have great memories when you are older.

If you try to attract a man who is a good father, who stays home with his family, works diligently at his job and showers you with gifts and attention, right now as a party girl, you'd go nuts. You'd think this type of man with stability traits, is boring.

Instead of trying to put a square peg in a round hole, answer these questions to attract Mr. Right now.

What do you bring to the relationship?
What type of person do you bring to the relationship? Who are you being? If you are being a fun-loving person, you'll attract someone who is looking for that quality.

If you are a quiet, reserved, caretaker, you'll attract someone who values those qualities. Make sure you are clear about what you like about yourself that you want your man to admire. This will ensure you attract a man who is right for you.

What do you enjoy doing?

Lots of advice books tell you to go where the men are. If you want to expose yourself to a new activity, that's good advice. But to show up at a sporting event looking cute, just to catch someone, will not serve you when he plans dates around these types of activities.

First of all, you won't be your best self because you are uncomfortable. Next, he will think he's found a soul mate based on a false belief. If you become a couple and he's willing to do things you enjoy and you are willing to compromise and do his stuff sometimes, the relationship could work.

But be ready with your list of what you really enjoy doing and be honest about it early in the relationship.

What do you value having?

If you value fast cars, and bling, be honest about it. A frugal man who wants a woman who values a white picket fenced home is not going to be pleased if you are really someone who wants the latest, most expensive trendy item.

The man who values your values is a better match. Make sure what you are collecting in your life reflects what you value.

How To Be Happy When You Have Nothing In Common

Happiness is the core reason we do anything. Think about it for a second, when you set any goal - even a goal to be happy when you have nothing in common with your man - why do you want the goal?

It's because whatever you will get out of that goal will make you happy won't it? And if you were happy all the time, would you really even need to have any goals?

When happiness is all a person ever really wants out of life in the end, then why would you want to put something of such great importance in the hands of another person?

True happiness is something that is best generated from

you. If you place your ability to be happy in something outside yourself, then your ability to be happy is never really in your control.

So when you think about how to be happy when you have nothing in common with your man, the real question is - "how can I just be happy?" - regardless of what my man interests are or what he is doing or even saying.

How can you be happy? This is a question you alone will need to discover within yourself. You must take some time to **get to know yourself and rediscover who you are** and what you truly like. Find the joy in everyday things.

If you are having trouble finding the joy in everyday life, consider changing the way that you look at things. Our perception of happiness is just that - a perception - a simple point of view. That simple point of view is A truth, but not the truth.

Being happy regardless of outside circumstances is a path worth seeking for the rest of your life. The moment you get it, then you are free - free from everything.

Don't wait for your man to change who they are. Don't wait for them to do something for you in order for you to be happy. Get your God given right to be happy now without having anything in common with your man.

If you discover that you need people who are like minded to share your life with, then seek them outside of your relationship or marriage. Life is too short to be miserable.

WHY MEN ARE SO CLUELESS WHEN IT COMES TO ONLINE DATING

Why do most men fail when it comes to online dating? Or feel that online dating has failed them? It's not their fault. They just don't understand online dating.

The reasons why there are so many people looking for a relationship on online dating websites are numerous. From being shy to wanting a quick bounce back after a breakup - all of this has made people turn to online dating and agencies.

Despite the fact that there are many people who have found what they have been looking for on one of the many dating websites, a lot of men still believe that this is not the way to start a relationship.

The reason why many men distrust online dating websites is that there are many misconceptions related to these websites.

Online Dating For Busy People
One of the biggest misconceptions on this subject is related to the question of who uses internet dating websites. Many men are of the opinion that these are the people who have a poor social life or cannot find a partner in "real life" due to the fact that they aren't physically attractive. This, however, couldn't be further from the truth.

The reasons why people create their profiles on internet dating sites are very different. One of the most common reasons for this is the busy schedule people have.

Owing to the fact that there are many people who are constantly snowed under by their work and don't have time to socialize, internet dating is one of the best solutions for them.

These websites are really well organized into several

categories such as dating for seniors, Christians or single parents. This makes it easy for people to find their match without having to waste a lot time.

Dating Websites for Finding True Love as Well as Just Having Fun

In this day and age, online dating is considered to be a good opportunity for people to find their true match and even get married. In the past, this wasn't the case.

The only people using these websites were insecure people or people who were desperate to find someone and afraid to be alone. This has made a lot of guys believe that it is not possible to find a partner using online dating websites.

What made most guys even more convinced in what they have previously believed are all those tips and advice on how to date as many women as you can.

This has brought up a question of why there is so much information on how to have a onetime thing if these websites were intended to help people find their true love. Well, these websites made for online dating aren't organized according to people's interests, age or beliefs only.

They are also organized based on what they expect from internet dating - whether they are looking for fun, adventure or they want to get married.

Men always think online dating websites are not efficient. The fact that more than one third of all marriages in the USA have started out as web dating only proves that these websites are efficient in helping people find their ideal partners.

Online dating websites give people the unique chance to meet a lot of people and choose their partners after they have met the most interesting and diverse people. Not until people realize this will they really know how amazing online dating can be.

How to Attract a Man

Online dating is a great way to meet men. Cute guys going through dry spells, shy boys who prefer to express themselves in writing, serious men who want to meet their future wives. There are tonnes of men out there with all kinds of direct or hidden agendas who would love to meet you.

The trick is to know what you want and how to attract a man who will give you exactly that. Stand out of the crowd of hundreds of women who are hopelessly waiting for Prince Charming to come around, and take your fate into your own hands.

There are many stories circulating about online dating, many about happy couples who met through these sites, but even more about the bitter disappointment of women who didn't find what they were looking for.

Why do you think that is? Some women might be too picky, others may jump into it with the wrong ideas, while many of them just probably don't understand the rules.

The first thing you should clarify when you register to an online dating site is what your purpose is. Are you looking for a relationship or will you be satisfied with a few fun dates with no strings attached?

It all depends on your goal. You will write one description about yourself if all you want is one hot steamy night, and whole different one for a possible boyfriend.

Write what you want them to read
Express yourself the way you want to be seen. This doesn't mean to write things which you wish were true but aren't, instead talk about all that is you, emphasizing the facts which set you apart from everyone else.

There's nothing attractive about a general description which could fit hundreds of women, so take the time and work that About Me page in your advantage. Omit things like your height and color of your eyes, instead linger on what you like about yourself and enjoy having it noticed. No one will know them if you don't write them down.

Also, casually mention what you're looking for, to avoid wasting your own precious time and of those who want something else. No need to talk about how many kids you prefer, but telling your potential readers that you expect more than a one night stand is a good idea.

Write what you want to read about

How are you going to attract a man who would share your interests if you don't mention what they are? Specify your hobbies and your accomplishments to wake the interest of fellow enthusiasts. If you could talk hours about your favorite film noir, this is a perfect way to find someone who wouldn't mind listening about it.

Write passionately about your "thing", may that be your award winning Chihuahua, your newly acquired vintage chopper, or your Poker skills. But don't turn your About Me page into an introduction to everything one needs to know about your hobby. I'm sure there are many things worth knowing about you, mention at least a few of them.

Remember: people who read about you don't know you. All they know is what you tell them in your online dating profile. How to attract a man who could be The One? Make sure he knows how great you are, and share some information by which you can connect.

THE MEANING OF THE "MALE EXPIRATION" DATE

What do you think? Do men have an expiry date? Do women? Do you think it's unfair that many people think women do and men don't?

Several men who, when they were young, had the world by

its tail. They were good-looking, successful, well-educated, well-traveled, lots of fun, with great personalities. They could have any woman they wanted.

And they wanted a lot of them. Usually, the party girls meaning very pretty but not very serious about life, the kind of girl you want to "date" but not marry.

Now that these men are older (mid 40's to late 40s), they want to find a nice woman, settle down and have a couple of kids. Here's the problem. Their value has fallen.

Now they are older, balding, had a profession that was extremely well paying back then but not really any more, one has an attitude of "I've had my fun, now it's time to have a family"- is he saying the good times are over and from here on out its watering the lawn and reading the paper?

Do you think it's realistic for these men to hope that they will find a woman young enough to bear children, that has everything going for her that they had going for them back in the day, and start a family with them from scratch?

The truth is when men don't have or have lost clear focus or direction or have not achieved success, something happens to their self esteem. They get a bashing. And when a man's ego is deflated, it can be mightily difficult being around him.

Of course, a man who has ambition can be mightily appealing - up to a point. And that point expires with his age. Stick around for long enough and, if he's done nothing, or hasn't reached his goals and he's still moping around in the belief that one day he is going to "make it", you'll be pulling out your own hair and might start wishing that you were a cougar instead ...

THE ONE AND ONLY "RULE" YOU NEED TO FOLLOW WHEN DATING MEN: MIRROR THEM

Did you know that there are certain ways to react to men, that will instantly make us like you more? Or that there are body language techniques you can use to make a man way more relaxed around you?

The thing is you are not all the time going to be fortunate in striking up a strong relationship with a man based on mutual tastes. The good news is there is a technique that you can use to produce the feeling of a bond. This technique is what psychologist call mirroring.

People who get on well with each other mirror each other naturally. The next time you're out on a date, and if you're wondering if your date likes you then just look at their body movements.

Notice if they are copying your none verbal communication if they are then the good news is you are probably on to a great relationship! So mirroring is just modeling another person's body language.

If you like a guy then you should try mirroring his gestures because that will send signals to his brain that you are in sync with him.

You can try this anywhere you wish whenever you spot a guy you wish to attract. There is high chance that you will catch a man's attention by simply mirroring his gestures. So use this little trick whenever you spot someone you like from afar and it will be a sure fire way to catch his attention and attract him to you.

Several extensive researches have been done on body language, and it has revealed some very interest information about reacting to body language. But before we get into that, let's quickly discuss the power of "similarity".

As you know, one of the keys to successful relationships in life is being similar to your partner. We generally like people who are similar to us. We like people with similar interests, similar taste in music, and similar experiences in life. If someone seems to be like us, then we automatically like them more.

Obviously then, anything we can do to make ourselves seem more similar to someone, will make them like us more. This great body language technique can make people like you more, without them even realizing it's happening.

Now, you have to get this right because there is definitely a right, and a wrong way, to mirror someone.

If you do it too much, it becomes too obvious. They will think you are mimicking them, and will not be impressed! You have to do it in a way that your man doesn't actually notice.

Suppose you are talking to a man, and you are both sitting at a table. During the conversation, he leans forward, and puts his hands on the table. When you notice this, wait about 45 seconds, and "mirror" his body language. i.e. You then lean forward, and put your hands on the table.

Later if he leans back, you wait around 45 seconds, and lean back as well. If he tilts his head, you do the same... about 45 seconds later.

Now, the timing doesn't have to be exactly 45 seconds! Don't start trying to count 45 seconds, or you will be too distracted. Just try and estimate when 30 seconds to a minute has gone past, and then mirror his movement.

This is an easy technique, but it's very powerful. And you can use it in all sorts of situations including in your love life. It works great on men. It's an all-round useful technique, that is great for making people subconsciously like you more.

Mirroring is a very clever seductive technique, comparable to hypnosis in its manipulative effectiveness. What better way to charm your way into a lover's heart then by stating, "I am so much like you...

I am your perfect mate!" Of course, no one will believe you if you tell them so outright. Mirroring is the subtle way of telling a person that you are their perfect complement.

Mirroring may involve very subtly mirroring your date's posture, their gestures and body language and even their personality and word usage. You cease becoming your own person and become who the other person is looking for.

You can't be too obvious about this technique or else your mirroring may be seen as mocking. Less is more in this regard. You can also mirror a person's vocal tones, their interests, and their appearance.

How to use mirroring to build relationships
Everyone has at one time or another taken something for granted. Possibly the thing that is taken for granted the most is your relationship. Hardly anyone ever stops to consider how re-lationships are formed, and how important they are - they are the core of everyone's happiness and future achievement.

A woman's capability to form connection with her man can make or break both their chances of happiness and success. The ability to create the right relationship is what gives a woman the advantage in relationship and other aspects of life.

When you begin to develop a relationship with someone the first thing you look for is similarity in personality. Most relation-ships are based on two people liking or disliking the same things. Same values and beliefs. Also the same interest in films, theatre and music etc.

When you use the technique of mirroring to build relation-ship with someone you need to make sure that you are doing it subtly. For instance if they do a gesture with their hands you could the do the same gesture a few seconds later.

Just don't do it at the same time, or they'll think that you are making fun of them. You can mirror a man by adopting a similar posture, laughing when he laughs and matching the pitch and tone of his voice.

Using Body Language - Secrets Guaranteed to Work

Have you always wondered how you can attract men using body language? Are you curious to see if you could use such simple gestures as a way to attract men?

I will tell you the ways that you can use your action to make men surround you. Attracting men is no easy feat and every aspect of our bodies can be used even our body language.

The way we move tells a lot about our personality and it also dictates the disposition the other person should be in when talking to you. Don't think that all men interpret body language right then and there but it is actually processed by the subconscious.

That is why it is important to make yourself be aware of how you move and use it to your advantage when you want to attract men.

Face value

The face is the guiding factor when dealing with body language. It is the first thing that welcomes or rejects a person from you. That is why it is never bad to keep a smile on your face and make men enticed to talk to you. Some women have this "auto-frown" facial expression that can make men walk away simply by the sight of the facial expression.

What the mirror tells us

Relationships is one area that people often ask about but lately it seems even more so. As the old is moving out and the new is moving in, we are shifting and so are our relationships. Women continually attracts unavailable men. Emotionally and physically unavailable, single and married men.

This has been a source of great frustration for most women as they are ready for a relationship and to share their lives with someone. So many attractive, smart, successful and creative women are not manifesting this relationship they desire?

Women get frustrated when they feel a connection to unavailable men repeatedly forgetting that men are a reflection of the type of person they are. You will keep attracting unavailable men because you are not available. Are you available?

THE VALUE IN LETTING A MAN CHOOSE YOU

Are You Choosing Someone Who Isn't Choosing You?

Why continue choosing into situations where you are not seen, valued or met?

At the beginning of any relationship there is some wooing that goes on. When you first start dating someone, it's natural to put a little more effort in so the other person knows that you like him.

But there is a line between wooing someone because you are mutually interested in relationship and convincing someone to be in a relationship with you.

Have you crossed the line? Here's how you know. When someone is clear - either in their words or behavior — that they are not looking for a commitment and you are, do you hear that information and know that it's your time to opt out because your values don't align?

Or do you fall in love with a fantasy? If someone continues to be slippery and not really act that into you, do you walk away or start to think of ways that you could possibly convince this person to pick you?

If you choose the latter, then you are entering into a future of senseless suffering. You will ignore your top values and instead listen to the voice of your ego, which says, "I want what I want and I'm going after it."

You then start thinking of ways to manipulate, convince and strategize your actions. At the same time, you will begin feeling rejected and obsessive.

As much as you say you want someone to be in a loving, intimate and committed relationship, part of you may not think it's possible. Maybe you've been hurt in the past by a committed relationship and unconsciously you are putting effort into a relationship that will never become committed as a way to protect yourself.

Or perhaps you have some limiting beliefs about your worthiness, which are fueling your pattern of chasing after crumbs. And as much as you want to receive love, there is something about it that scares you. Or even worse, thinks you don't deserve it.

If this resonates with you, invest the energy that you are investing in chasing after a slippery person into yourself. Heal your wounds and update your beliefs. Make creating a healthy relationship with you the object of your desire.

Are you waiting to be chosen?

When people explain their frustrations with dating or how they're feeling rejected after a possible date didn't materialize, or not getting past a date or few with someone, what I realize is some of you are waiting to be chosen.

In these situations, the dynamic is imbalanced from the outset because you're putting your fate into someone else's hands, because you assume that if they choose you that it's something you want to be in, and on the flipside you assume that if you're not chosen that it must definitely have been a relationship you should have had.

The trouble with all of this is you're not showing up as someone who is holding their own and owning their right to choose and go through the discovery phase of dating. Instead, you're taking a more passive role where you're happy to be the passenger on whatever journey the driver takes you on, just as long as they take you on a journey and keep driving.

If 'chosen' for their journey, you may be happy to make their agenda your agenda, or you will privately decide that when you've got your feet well and truly under the proverbial table, that you'll be so valued and loved, that they'll be willing to change.

In effect, it's like handing over a Choose Me Stick – when someone is in possession of it, they have the power to choose you, validate you, and even shape you.

Why? Because when you're not showing up to your dates and relationships as an equal party with your eyes and ears open with the right to choose, the only choice you have is to subconsciously and possibly even consciously adapt your behaviour to increase the chances of being chosen.

Think about it: While it's very possible that initially you might be yourself, as soon as you start to feel like they're 'pulling away', or you've already stuck your pump on them and started inflating who they are so that you can think that they're way more special than they are while they look down on you from that pedestal.

If what's on your mind is to be chosen, then you're going to reflect that in your behaviour which essentially boils down to being and doing things that contradict your values to hold onto someone you haven't positively chosen, at all costs.

Whatever it is, you change, morph, adapt, twist, and contort to be chosen. You also go into a holding pattern circling over the possibility of the relationship that you want, hoping that air traffic control will give you the signal that you can land and take up your slot.

Waiting for someone to make you a priority, to proceed to a relationship, to not breakup, to leave a different partner, or whatever it is that you're waiting to be chosen for, just de-prioritizes you.

If you prioritized you, you'd never be in a situation where someone not only has the power to decide your fate, but to leave a crater sized hole in your life, because by handing out so much power, you're bound to feel very rejected when it all goes tits up.

When you're not co-choosing in a mutually beneficial relationship, it all becomes about one person working harder than the other, which by default assigns greater 'value' - they're just not that special.

You may go for the easy, low-hanging fruit option and choose people that you perceive as being more likely to be with you. It could be that you recognize certain things that would register as issues to avoid with someone else, but you see it as an opportunity. Of course, when it doesn't pan out, it's like "I can't believe someone like them doesn't want me - what's wrong with me?"

Or you will choose a challenge in the form of someone who you think is unlikely to choose you, which may be simply based on the fact that you'd have to convince them to make you the exception to their rule of being unavailable.

Waiting to be chosen is a bit like how some people go about job hunting – they put so much energy into being the right person for the job, it's assumed that it's the right job for them.

Interview processes do actually involve you evaluating whether it's the right job for you, which will arise from the questions you ask and what you glean during the interview process plus any other research you do.

Instead they get the job offer and then start evaluating whether it's actually the right opportunity for them. If they don't get the job, some take it as a huge blow of rejection.

Of course it's not as great an issue with your job hunting unless you end up miserable in a job that you knew wasn't right for you but felt compelled to take it because you were asked, or you feel blah about your career, or you end up floating around getting job offers but never staying in a job for any decent length of time and always have a foot out the door...

With dating and relationships, once you start dipping into

the Illusions Account, the High Growth Sexual Activity Fund and start planning a future around this idea of what it'll be like to be The Chosen One, you can see why you will struggle to deal with rejection.

You don't spend enough time asking if it's the right job for you, just like you don't ask if it's the right relationship for you. It's like there's a job going that's in your field - you want it.

Someone in your common interests, appearance or whatever 'field' has a vacancy, you're on it without even truly evaluating what the 'opportunity' is. "I'm on it! I'm on it!"

You're just not that desperate. You technically have a 'vacancy' too - surely you don't want to give it to any 'ole Muppet off the street?

One of the things that job interviews and eventually dating and relationships taught me, is that anything that you get 'rejected' by through the process of not being 'chosen', there's normally a very good reason why you wouldn't have chosen them either.

The overwhelming majority of the time, you are already aware of these reasons, it's just that you get sidetracked by your ego that needs that gold star of someone choosing you. It's like "I want to be chosen so I have the option of telling them to bog off."

Understanding Men In Relationships

Many women feel they just don't get men and how they think in relationships. If there is a basic misunderstanding, there are bound to be problems that arise. Here are a few simple tips to help you deal better with the opposite sex.

Here are 7 good tips:
1- Don't beat around the bush

Speak your mind clearly. Say what you mean and mean what you say. Though some are into game playing, they are not mind readers. If an issue needs addressed, address it and cut-to-the chase.

2- Basic Grooming

If your man seems to have forgotten basic grooming or has some other annoying habit that he has allowed to resurface, a gentle reminder should do the trick. Don't nag. It won't get you to your desired goal anyway.

Perhaps he has forgotten he should open the door for you. You may try a little cough or a simple gesture towards the door.

3- Ask for compliments

If you want him to compliment you and he doesn't, just ask. Asking for compliments is also to see if he your choice of style and color, etc. A little flattery and suggestion of coloring and styling for your guy is acceptable, too. Yes, we do like compliments too.

4- Men are used to being the ones to ask someone out

So if there's a place you want to go, make sure to bring it up. And don't be afraid or timid about speaking up to voice your opinions about what you want, where you want to go, what you want to eat, etc.

Especially in the world of dieting today, males tend to think that all females are dieting and want salads for meals. If you have an appetite for seafood and steak - speak up!

5- Don't play games

It is OK to flirt and tease a little bit. Men even expect you to do it some. But do not become a game player. It is an easy way to go from being interesting to not being taken seriously at all.

6- Establish rapport with the man in your life

It is fairly easy to get into rapport with a person when there is a common interest. If you both like each other, that is motivation enough to begin to mirror and match his motions and gestures. Ladies, this technique works and works well with someone you just met.

Now don't be so obvious with it, but when he makes a hand gesture, you follow with a similar hand gesture. If his voice tone is lower and conversational, adjust your volume to match his.

If your man is being romantic over dinner, you do not want your laughter to be loud! Understand? Mirror and match him and watch the sparks fly.

7- Become interested in what he is interested in

That does not mean you have to become an expert in football or soccer. But you can take an interest in his hobbies and learn the basics. He will appreciate you taking the time to enter his world so to speak.

It may make him a little more willing to listen to you yammer on and on about the new shoes and purse you just bought. You need to just remember this: Smart is sexy. Uninformed and dumb is. ...well you already know the answer to that one.

WHEN YOU SHOULD SLEEP WITH A GUY – AND HOW TO STALL EFFECTIVELY UNTIL YOU KNOW HE'S BOYFRIEND MATERIAL

Sleeping with a man isn't always the event of the century, but very few women ever master the technique of 'casual sex'.

In fact, most women expect to feel nothing after the fact, but that's simply not the case most of the time - especially if they like the man they slept with and see some potential relationship material when they stare at him in the morning before he wakes up.

The sad but honest truth is that even though a man is into you sexually, it doesn't automatically mean he's into you in any other way.

Women often expect more once they devote themselves intimately - whether they consciously think so or not - and sometimes, men don't get more interested but less, and start to "cool off" and act distant when all the woman wants is an even deeper connection.

A situation happening this way is pretty common, and usually it doesn't make any lady feel good about herself and her decision to sleep with a man. So to avoid such self-esteem crushing feelings, it's important to be aware of exactly what you should know before you take a handsome hunk to bed.

Intimate connection isn't always the beginning of a relationship. It's hard to separate all the feelings out when you feel sparks fly, especially when you haven't had that kind of connection in awhile.

And just because you both feel that way about one another doesn't mean that you both interpret that feeling in the same way, since men and women are different in the way they view relationships much of the time.

Even when a man spends time with you and seeks you out via phone and text and makes out with you in the broom closet doesn't mean he necessarily wants a relationship with you.

If your new man is sending you mixed messages, sometimes it's best to just ask what he expects out of the relationship before it gets too deep on your end. You may not like the answer, but it's better to know now rather than later when you've already fallen head over heels and he's still skirting around the edges of what could be a relationship.

Sex will never help a man "see your worth". Sex is fun, and it can bring out the best sensuality and romance in people, but it will never be the same as a man's respect. The desire to have sex in its very basic form will usually stem from a very pure attraction to another person.

It may be pheromones, or maybe your new guy likes blondes, but physical desire and attraction doesn't usually mean anything more than just that. It doesn't mean that the guy likes your personality, and it definitely doesn't help them understand what a wonderful person you are, or what you're like outside the bedroom.

This may seem a little over the top for you, but asking yourself "does this man value me for the strong, interesting, amazing woman that I am?" before you sleep with a man, you may determine if sleeping with him will put you on unequal terms and understanding of what's going on.

We don't fall in love with you because you're good in the bedroom. When you feel an intense physical and emotional connection with a man, usually have at least a hint of emotional connection with him once the night is over.

With time, this connection can get stronger and more intimate, making it even more challenging to deal with the aloofness of the man you slept with who obviously doesn't feel the same way.

Sleeping with a guy doesn't mean he's going to become more connected with you in any way other than sexually. A man's love will usually come over time as he realizes you're something special and he wants to keep you in his life.

Sometimes this happens off the bat, but it's rare at best. Long term love usually takes long term commitment and patience, and that's exactly what you should expect.

Don't sleep with a man unless you're absolutely sure you are both on the same level. Know yourself - and know that you probably will feel closer and more interested in your man after you have sex with him, and he may not feel the same way and usually won't for a long while.

Sleep with him when you're both ready to commit to trying something out and you've talked about it, and the right man will wait until you've worked everything out in your own head before involving him - if he leaves, then he just wasn't right for what you need.

Is it a good idea to put off sex with your guy?

How do you tell if it's time to sleep with your new boyfriend, or if you should put off sex until a later date? Do you ever worry that you will ruin your relationship by getting him in the sack too soon?

How do you know if he's really into you, or just looking for sex? You're not the only woman to ponder these questions. The answers are all very good reasons to put off having sex with your new guy until you know how the relationship is shaping up.

Is he in it for the sex?

Simply put, men sometimes use women for sex. This is not to say that every guy just wants in your pants and nothing else. But there are those men who have no intention of getting serious with you, no matter what the two of you get up to in bed.

You need to know whether your new crush is one of these or not, otherwise you could end up feeling hurt and used. The good news is that when a man is truly in to you, he won't mind waiting. In fact, lots of men prefer to take things slower when they feel they've found someone special.

How will sex affect your relationship?

Women tend to attach emotions to sex, while men do not. To you, sleeping together may feel like an intensely emotional experience that strengthens the bond between you.

To him, he may feel as if he just got laid and nothing else. This will leave the two of you on different wavelengths regarding the relationship. You will have moved on to the next stage while he has not.

Will he think you're cheap?

A good reason to put off sex until you two get to know one another is that it makes you look classy, not cheap. Even if you're both heavily infatuated and you know sleeping together would be a good experience, doing the deed too early in a relationship can give him the wrong impression.

He may wonder if you treat all your dates to the privileges he's getting, or he may mistakenly believe you just wanted a one-night stand.

The temptation to sleep with a guy early on in a relationship can be overwhelming, especially if you've had your eye on him for a long time, or if you believe he's really in tune with your needs.

But think before you act. If you can restrain your urges and put off sex until the two of you are more familiar with each other, it will allow the real, emotional side of the relationship to develop. And it will make the night that you do get busy a very special and exciting one.

Did you sleep with a guy too soon? How to undo the damage and regain his interest

Lust can lead us to do things we later regret. Many women have experienced this and quite often the thing they do is they sleep with a guy too soon. We all know the unspoken rule of waiting a few dates before getting intimate with a new guy.

Building the anticipation and keeping some mystery about you will usually help to capture his long term attention. If you've already made the mistake and now he seems completely disinterested in you, take heart.

There is a way you can undo the damage and make him chase after you just as aggressively as he did before you two had sex.

Obviously if you did sleep with a guy too soon you can't turn back the hands of time. You have to accept that it's happened and the only place to go is forward. You don't get a do-over on this. The deed has been done and it's time to look to the future.

If he's starting to call less often or if he comes up with excuses for why he can't see you, he's definitely starting to lose interest.

One crucial mistake that many women make after they do this is they decide they need to explain themselves to the man in question.

They believe that if they tell him that they aren't normally like that or that they've never slept with another man so early in the relationship that he'll forget all about it. He won't. In fact, he'll think you're putting too much effort into trying to undo it.

One easy way to get that back is to take the romantic aspect of the relationship out of the equation, for now. Often, when a woman sleeps with a man too early he thinks she wants a commitment.

He'll pull back because he's scared of that. Show him that you're just as happy to be his friend. Ask him out for lunch or a coffee. Don't chase him down trying to line up some evening plans with him. Give him a little space but let him know you're still available, but not to sleep with.

The best thing you can do if you sleep with a guy too soon is pull back from him a bit. He's likely already doing this with you and you need to follow suit.

A great piece of advice that often works for women in this situation is to approach him from a place of friendship rather than one of romance. Shift your train of thought towards building a solid friendship with him.

If you two are still going out, you're probably wondering how you should handle intimacy with him. If you slept with him too soon your initial reaction may be to pull back completely and not sleep with him again right now.

If you do that he'll wonder what is going on with you. The key is to time intimacy carefully and make sure it's not the sole focus of your relationship. Make plans to go out sometimes and then don't stay over at his place and don't invite him over to yours.

Make it clear, through your actions, that you're not there just to have sex with him. There is a delicate balance to this though as you don't want him to think that you've lost all interest in him as a lover.

Ensure he sees that you're fun in every setting. Plan outings and activities that keep you away from the bedroom for awhile. If you're out having fun together and sex isn't an option he'll start to see all facets of you.

That's when you'll be able to really pique his interest. You'll have him wanting you in more ways than one.

Playing Hard To Get Until You Are Sure He's A Good Material
Do you know you should be playing hard to get? Do you know how? Do you try so hard? Do you want to become an arch seduc-

tress? If you have a hard time getting to date the men you really want then you need to learn the secrets...

You may have heard the old cliché "treat them mean to make them keen", and, sure it's a cliché, but that's because there is some truth in it. You know in your heart of hearts that a man can soon lose interest in a girl who is too "easy". A man does not think something is worthwhile unless he has put in some effort.

Being mean in this context does not imply being downright rude or cantankerous, but simply means showing that you have personality and a mind of your own. You do not want to necessarily always agree with everything he says for example.

A woman with some knowledge and her own views on current events, politics or music is a much more interesting prospect. You don't need to bend to his will straightaway or be always available for him. By maintaining a slight air of mystery you increase his interest in you.

This is an art that comes naturally to some women but if you're the straightforward type you may have to practice a little bit.

Think of playing hard to get as a game that will make the relationship more exciting for both of you, and, a slight unpredictability in a women is a quality guaranteed to keep a man's interest. He will not get bored if he can't read your mind and doesn't know what you will do or say next.

Playing hard to get is a little like walking a tightrope in that if you should make a mistake you may have blown it. If you make it too difficult for the guy to date you he may eventually give up.

As a rule of thumb a chap who is snubbed more than twice might not bother to ask you a third time. It's partly a matter of course how you handle his offer to take you out.

You do not want to turn him down flat but rather decline

gracefully with the intimation that you would consider it but this particular time is not convenient.

By making out how busy your social life is you are a more attractive proposition and he can see that he will have to put in some effort to win you over.

When you are on a date with a guy that you're keen on you will obviously want to be fun and enthusiastic. Treat him like he's the most important person in the world, giving him your full attention. This will get his attention since men love flattery as much as women.

When you are apart from him, do make sure you have other things in your life. Get on with your life without dwelling on the relationship and how it's going. Too much analysis can kill the fun and spontaneity in a relationship.

When you see him next don't say you have missed him as you don't want to give away too much too soon. If a guy thinks he's all ready "cracked it" he is less likely to try hard to please you and he may become bored or boring.

The ideal situation is to keep a guy interested but guessing. Don't ramble on about what you have been doing unless he specifically asks, and, even then be a little vague. This will stir up his interest and make him want to spend more time with you and get to know more about you.

If you manage this then you have become the seductress, the victor in the dating game. You know the secret of getting a man to want you and to chase after you to gain your favour.

Clever Tricks To Keep Him Hooked
One of the best tips on how to play hard to get is giving your guy a challenge. Be a little difficult. There's something very intriguing about a woman that's feisty and hard to get. But be careful though because while playing hard to get will keep a man interested, it's also a game wherein you can lose your man if you

make the wrong move.

Learn how to play hard to get the right way with these tips so you wouldn't end up losing your man.

• Don't immediately return his calls. Wait at least a day before you call him back. But be sure not to make him wait for too long. Keeping him waiting for a day will make him wonder about you.

• Unless it's an important message, don't respond to his emails or messages. If you should reply, wait a couple of days before you do. This will make you look busy and hard to get, so he has to work extra hard if he wants to get your attention.

• Be bold and ask him to hang out, but add a little twist: only do this when you have other friends around. Asking him to do something alone with you screams you're interested in him, so just ask him to join you and your friends. It's also a great way for him to get to know your clique.

• If you think he's going to ask you out, make it seem that your schedule is packed. If he asks "what are you doing this Saturday", say "I'm not sure yet." Then tell him you may be able to squeeze in a few hours for him.

• One great advice on how to play hard to get is to enjoy your single life. Love comes when you least expect it, and when you just enjoy yourself, playing hard to get comes naturally. A busy person is more attractive because you're naturally a challenge because you're unavailable most of the time. Beats being bored and waiting around.

HOW TO READ A MAN'S MIND
AND KNOW IF HE IS LYING

Do you know how to read a man's mind? Can you tell what your man is thinking at any given moment? Can you really say with some form of certainty that you can correctly predict how your man will behave given certain conditions and circumstances? Well very few people can answer these questions with certainty.

To be able to have a relationship that is of high value, you need to be able to read your man at least to some extent. You need to know if he really likes you, if he is into you well enough to make you the one.

Your man may be the silent type, too silent to the point that you constantly have to guess what exactly is going on in his mind. You do not always have to **force him to talk** as there are alternative means to get him to talk. When you want to look deeper into your man's mind, here are some tips that you could follow:

Learn how to read his facial expression...
Your man isn't that good an actor to always have a poker face. Make sure you know what is going on in his mind by reading how he reacts to things that you say.

Decipher the words that he uses.
To know how to read a man you can also find out what he is thinking about through his choice of words. To know how to read a man's mind, you must know his facial expressions, some context clues would also tell you exactly how he feels. For instance, you can mention the word **commitment**, then ask him about it. Listen to the adjectives that he'd use to describe the word commitment.

His eyes are the windows to his soul.

Even if your man is trying to pacify you and is trying to convince you that he'll marry you, if his eyes tell otherwise, then you have to believe what his eyes tell. Look into a man's eyes when he's trying to tell you something. When he twitches or fidgets as he can't even look you straight in the eye, then he's definitely lying about something.

Get vital information from his friends.

To know how to read a man's mind, his friends may be an excellent source of information because there may be some things that your man might tell them but is hesitant to tell you. If you've gained favor in their sight before, then fishing for some information is no gargantuan task for you.

Check his online blogs (if he has any).

A lot of people now do some blogging and online journals are the hottest trends these days. You would be truly lucky if your man has one. Get to know your man and the things that are going on in his head through his writings. You may feel like a stalker at first, but it's alright. Treat the situation like you're just a normal reader and you just want to get to know him more.

Let him be caught off guard.

If you want to know the truth, you can try talking to your man when he least expects you to. Surprise him by mentioning the word commitment out of the blue. The element of surprise would surely make him blurt out the exact feelings that he has.

Use a time-tested scheme.

If you want to know his true feelings, try to come up with something unique. For instance, use a third party. Tell him that your friend is asking advice from you, when the truth is the "friend" is really you. Get him to say what he really thinks about any issue.

How to Know If He Is Lying

Looking for the lie or like in so many relationships "the lies". But how do you know that he is indeed lying, without raising hell and being called paranoid, jealous, and stupid and the multitude of other insults that he conjures up when you dare to speak your mind about his unacceptable behavior

I know how crazy it feels to wonder if the man you love is trust-worthy. So here are 3 ways that I use to know how to tell if your Man is lying...

1. He gets defensive and starts to attack you

If he says things like "You are being too suspicious.", "How can you not trust me?", "Stop trying to control me", consider them warning bells.

A good Man, who is serious about you, will do his best to reassure you, instead of making you guilty for **asking him questions** about his location, his activities, his friends, etc. There is no good reason for your boyfriend to make you feel bad if he is not lying about something.

Even if he is not lying about where is, who he's meeting or what he's doing, he could be lying about his desire to be in a committed relationship with you. Because... if he were truly interested about being your boyfriend, he would take care of your feelings. He would not attack you if he were truly into you.

2. After listening to his explanation, for some reason, you still don't believe him

If your Man gives you a logical and rational **explanation to your questions**, and you still don't feel right, this is your intuition talking. You feel what you feel, and you can choose to either listen or ignore your intuitive feelings. I've learnt the hard way that my feelings are my friend, and that I should trust them.

The way you feel is part of you. If you stand up for your feelings, and let your boyfriend tell you that your feelings are wrong, you start to lose an important part of who you are. So who do you trust? Your own feelings that have accompanied you your whole life, or your boyfriend whom you've known for a much shorter time?

3. His story doesn't match up when you check up on him

For example, he says he's going out with his friends, but when you call to ask what they're doing, he doesn't describe much to you. If your Man is serious about being in a relationship with you, he will be eager to prove himself to you. That is why, **you need to ask your boyfriend** for his friends' names, and continue to ask him to tell you more about them.

A good Man will be keen to tell you more about his friends. More than that, he will be eager for you to meet his friends. Also, when you ask him whether you can join their gathering, he will either agree or give you a satisfactory explanation about why it's not a good idea.

To summarize, how to read a man's mind to know if your Man is lying is to ask him questions, listen to what your intuitive feelings tell you, and be aware that he won't need to attack your behaviour if he has nothing to hide.

UNDERSTANDING THE COMMITMENT PHOBIA AND WHY MEN ARE AFRAID TO COMMIT

What exactly is commitment phobia?

For most people, keeping relationships come naturally. However, there are some who find it quite a challenge. These people feel anxious when it comes to making a commitment with someone. Commitment phobia is based on anxiety and fear – they are afraid that things won't go right for them when they stay in one long-term relationship.

You need to understand that people with commitment phobia are capable of loving people but their feelings can be very powerful and they may feel an intense fear.

In the beginning of a relationship, they may enjoy feelings of intimacy and affection, but the anxiety increases as the relationship goes on. Then when expectations of commitment are expressed, or implied, the fear multiplies and the person tries to get out of it.

Don't take it personally – a person with commitment phobia really does want to stay with another person he loves, but their fear is often overwhelming so they would rather stay away from it. Even if they do agree to be in a commitment, they might back away after some time because they can't calm their fears.

Many times, commitment-phobes often come from backgrounds where one parent walked out on the family, and so as children, perhaps they develop a fear that such actions and choices are hereditary, that the tendency to walk out is passed down from parent to child and they, too, are doomed to repeat the same actions.

Or, they may know it's not hereditary, but they don't want to repeat—consciously or unconsciously--the same actions as the parent who abandoned them. So, they may get close to someone for a while, but back off as soon as things just start to get good, or perhaps not engage in romantic relationships of any substance at all, and have countless one-night-stands that provide little in the way of a solid relationship because they don't want to get involved enough to either get hurt, or hurt someone else.

Also, commitment-shy men might simply have been badly burnt by a previous relationship where the women in their lives tried to control and monitor their actions, and they want nothing to do with commitment after that because they do not want a repeat of the same. Who can blame them, right? After all, no one wants to be controlled like that.

It is important for people with commitment issues to recognize their feelings so that they do not confuse excitement, joy, and anticipation with anxiety and fear.

It is easy to confuse these emotions as it is said that chemically speaking, the chemicals for fear and the chemicals for joy, excitement and anticipation are quite similar. People who are afraid of commitment want to keep their freedom and individuality—the fears of losing such being rooted in controlling relationships of the past---while they also desire intimacy and exclusivity.

Understanding Fears

You need to understand that his fear of commitment is rooted on several other fears. This apprehension, as mentioned before, can be the result of a desire to keep one's independence and individuality or from past experiences and relationships.

1. Fear of Rejection

Men who have previously experienced rejection do not want to suffer it again. Even if they feel so strongly for a woman, they worry because that person may not love him back the same way.

Or that person may love him but not deeply enough to the point of sticking around and being there for him. Hurt feelings from past rejection can cause a man to hold back in investing his emotions.

While this is talking about men, women can experience the same stuff. They can also experience the feeling of worry about not being loved back, so even women can experience a good deal of commitment-phobia.

2. Fear of Failure

Since committing yourself to someone involves responsibilities, there will be expectations. Some men don't want to be burdened with these expectations because they fear that they might fail.

All men have this desire to excel, and with the thought of missing the mark and disappointing their partner in the future, they would rather avoid commitment.

This fear of failure in a man might also be rooted in watching his female relatives being super-snooty, picky and complaining to their menfolk that "this isn't right" or "that isn't right," or whatever else they're kvetching about.

Such talk would make anyone feel awful about themselves, but men can really take this to heart to the point of not even wanting to commit to the women they've fallen for, because they might be afraid the women are going to turn "shrewish."

3. Longing for Independence

Boys grow up to be men who desire to be independent. They don't like to rely on somebody else, specifically a woman. Some men think that when they commit to someone, they will end up depending on them completely. This perspective keeps them from getting into commitments.

However, this is probably perfectly understandable from your view, since many modern women want grown-up independent men who don't constantly need looking after.

They want a guy who's engaged with his feelings, but they don't want an emotionally co-dependent and overly needy man, either, because otherwise, it's like raising a son instead of being married to a full-grown man.

4. Fear of Change

Not everyone likes change. Committing to someone in a relationship will mean that you will change your life and your ways. It will no longer be about you – but about the other person, too.

Often, men are comfortable with what they already have and since they are unsure of the future, they will not move forward and just hold on to what they presently have and do.

The thing to remember about fear is that it's an old primal response to threats to the status quo. If all is not quiet "on the western front," when it comes to life's turbulence, for good or ill, a man's instinctive urge is to make sure things go back to the way they were before the "turbulence" started.

They don't know how to adjust to "a new normal," even if they want you to be part of that "new normal." Other men may want the change, but still become fearful that the "bubble will burst," that you will leave.

So, they do what they can to keep the bubble from bursting and just not engage in commitment to begin with. But this still keeps them unsatisfied, so they keep repeating this cycle ad nauseum. At least until they figure out how to break the cycle and move forward past the fear.

5. Inability to Share Life

There are men who are largely committed to their own lives and what they have made of it. These can be men who are highly successful, financially secure and at the peak of their careers. The problem with these men is that they are not eager to share their success.

They are afraid that their partners will take advantage of them once they are committed. This could be because they've experienced "gold-diggers" before: the types of women who could not see the men as they are, but instead saw what hooking up to a wealthy man can get them in life, without giving back.

6. Fear of Changing Their Identity

While there are men who fear that the individual lives they have created will change, they are also afraid that their identities will be altered. For instance, a man may think that he will become this image—essentially become a person he doesn't recognize as himself--once he gets married or committed to a single person.

When he doesn't like that projection, he will not enter into a commitment. Such a man's fear is understandable, but it may take some time for them to be convinced that just because you get married doesn't mean you must give up your identity, your core nature as a human individual.

Yes, couples do end up influencing each other as far as habits are concerned, big or small, because the longer we are with a person, our auras mesh together, and our habits rub off on each other via familiarity.

It has even been said that we retain part of another's auric essence when merging energies during sexual intercourse, but that's a topic for another time.

7. Keeping Options Available

Men who don't want to commit are often thinking of somebody else. They fear that somebody better than the woman they have may come along and they will miss the opportunity, so they choose not to settle down.

But remember—even the most well-known "eternal bachelor" George Clooney found the one woman who made him realize she was the right one for him and finally got married.

Why Men Are Afraid to Commit

While there are women who are also commitment phobic, this fear is more common to men. Here are some of the common reasons why men are afraid to commit or don't even think about it:

1. He doesn't believe in exclusivity

That guy still likes to play the field – meaning, he still wants to date other women. By making a commitment, he will lose the right to do so and he does not like that. Often, a man will try to cling to this right for as long as he can. This is especially true of a young man when he is not yet sure what he is looking for in a woman.

Hopefully, you'll meet up with a guy who's honest enough about this during the dating process so you won't get your heart completely broken. Well, you might at least be disappointed—especially if he's a decent enough guy overall.

But if he's honest about his not being ready to settle down, you can say "sayonara" as peaceably as you can and move on to the next guy without a lot of emotional investment.

2. He is not matured enough – or doesn't want to grow up

For men, commitment means maturity. It means they will "grow up" – and they don't like that. They want to be young and free. They want to be able to do what they like without the accompanying responsibilities.

They will delay this process as much as they can. Clearly, if you know guys like this, it's kind of obvious you don't want to tangle with them if you're thinking marriage.

3. He is already committed

The man who is afraid to commit may already be committed to somebody else, at least in his mind. For example, a past relationship. This is the man who has a problem letting go of his previous commitment and doesn't want to be involved with somebody else in the same level.

This can apply to men whose girlfriends have just broken up with them, or perhaps they are widowers who are still grieving long after their wife has passed from this earthly life.

They cannot imagine being with any other woman. While this devotion can seem sweet, it can be heart-crushing for you if you are sweet on the man in question and his heart is still not available, even though he lives alone.

4. He has his own timetable – he is not sure of it

If he's going to come around, it will be when he's ready, not on your timetable. He really doesn't know when or if he'll ever be ready for the commitment you're looking for. In which case, you might want to review your own timetable and see if you're not being too strict about having things go your way.

Many women do this: they think they must graduate college by 21, get their Master's Degree by 26, marry by 30 (no later than! Biological clock, you know!), have the requisite old-school "white-picket-fence-nuclear-family" number of 2.5 kids, a dog, cat and a gerbil by 34, and on and on; their lives are planned to the nth degree, leaving no room for actual life, or other people's journeys to actually matter.

You may be in love with an easy-going guy because he's not like you, and you may find that your easy-going guy may want to commit, but if you are so dead-set on controlling your life, and your timetable is so planned out that there is no room for him to make his own decisions, he may very well refuse to commit—and maybe even say "au revoir" before you even have a chance to deliver some crazy ultimatum.

Especially if he doesn't like the idea of you being so controlling. There is a big difference between lovingly requesting a solid commitment from a guy overall, and demanding he commit to you according to your own timetable, and not allow him to have his own decisions about his life.

5. He thinks the timing isn't right

Some men don't want to take their relationships to the next level because they feel that they need to focus on themselves.

Men in college, for instance, who want to concentrate on getting a job, or those who want to impress their bosses and co-workers because they are eyeing promotions. They know that work may take its toll on their time and energies so they don't want the burden of handling a relationship.

They don't necessarily like to mess around with other girls while they are dating someone, but they don't want to have that extra worry when they are out in the bar with friends. He wants to give his 100% in the relationship but he cannot at the moment, so he would rather not commit until then.

If this is the case, then you have every right to break things off and go do your own thing. If he wises up and realizes you're the woman for him after all this time, he will come seek you out. If he doesn't, then he clearly was not the man for you after all, and you are still free to date someone who is a little more settled and sure of his journey in life.

6. His past experiences with a present girlfriend or with an ex makes him hesitant

There are things women do that men hate. Sometimes, they don't say it, but deep down, it bothers them and turns them off.

It can be something that happened in a past relationship or something that is currently happening – it keeps a man from committing because he fears that things won't change for the better or these red flags might become worse and he can't handle it.

A mature man, however, is going to eventually find his voice and speak of these annoying things in a rational way, at least as best he can, instead of being passive-aggressive and just stewing about it.

After all, if you are in a relationship with a man and you are not just lovers but good friends, he is going to want to clear the air with you if he wants a commitment. Plus, true friends don't let each other get away with BS—and that includes friends who are also lovers.

If something you do bothers your man, and he has the maturity to be rational, yet the courage to speak his mind about those things that tick him off, and the willingness to work things out, then you've got a keeper when it comes to commitment.

You will meet commitment phobes – or those who have commitment issues – in all shapes, sizes and behaviors. These people's view of relationships and their patterns vary.

There are some who will not have a serious relationship that will last longer than a week, while there are others who may commit for a few months but do not last long term because their fears come up and they either leave or drive their partner away.

If you want to have lasting, meaningful relationships, then you need to overcome the fear of commitment. Madeleine L'Engle so aptly puts it this way, "If we commit ourselves to one person for life, this is not, as many people think, a rejection of freedom; rather, it demands the courage to move into all the risks of freedom, and the risk of love which is permanent; into that love which is not possession but participation."

To continue Madeleine L'Engle's line of thinking, when we commit to one person, we put down roots and we Deepen. Meaning we end up realizing there is more to marriage than just the nuts and bolts, the comings and goings of everyday life.

We get to grow spiritually with the other person. We get to be witness to each other's life journey, to see each other through the rough parts, laugh during the good ones, and enjoy all the other moments in between.

And to do this, it takes a lot of trust on our parts, make no mistake about that. It takes a lot of trust to open our hearts to another person, for them to know us and our souls intimately, and to learn even more about each other as we grow and change and Deepen individually.

Commitment's not just something you say you're going to embark on just because everyone says it's a good thing. In truth, commitment to just one other person is a privilege. All the more reason to make the kind of choices that lead us to the right person to share that privilege with.

7 WAYS TO TRIGGER THE COMMITMENT INSTINCT IN YOUR MAN

Are you finding it hard to make your man show some commitment in your relationship? Perhaps you are looking for an easy way to trigger the commitment instinct in your man? Most men are afraid of commitments and this has created a bad impression about the unserious approach of men to relationships.

Definition of Commitment In A Relationship

Before we go further, the question really is; what is commitment in relationships? Let's define commitment in relationships. Commitment in a relationship means the final decision from each of both partners to dedicate and give their all into the success of the relationship.

Have you found that type of guy that sweeps you off your feet with just a smile? Do you wish to experience the commitment love with him? But all you see is the fear of commitment relationship.

Is your heart telling you to do one thing contrary to your expert's view? It is a difficult decision when faced with commitment relationship issues. However, this article is aimed at unleashing different working ways by which you can trigger the commitment instinct in your man.

This of course will lead to you and your spouse having a wonderful commitment dating experience.

Understand Male Psychology

Male and female are entirely two different being. You need to have an understanding of the male psychology. You need to know when he falls in love with you. You need to understand how a man acts when he's falling in love with you.

You need to put in some hard work to understand the way he thinks. You can start by giving answers to these questions!

- How does a man act when he's falling in love?
- What makes a man fall in love psychologically?
- What makes a man love a woman forever?
- What makes a man fall in love and stay in love?

All these and some other few male psychological questions are very important questions you need to answer.

Be A High Value Woman

Men are logical being so they tend to see things the direct and logical way. They are able to figure out and differentiate between confidence and low self-esteem.

This is why you need to create value for yourself by being a high value woman. So, what is a high value woman? A high value woman is one who knows what she wants, goes for it and never lowers her standard.

She is strong, independent and confident of herself. She says "no" and means it. This attribute comes in form of challenge for men and as we all know, men are moved by challenges. This would surely ignite his commitment instinct.

Make Him Need You

There are various ways to which you can get a guy committed to you but none beats making him need you. This strategy is guaranteed to make you end up being the one for him.

Naturally, men love the chase, the challenge, and they tend to get more attracted to women they find it hard to get. Now, you have to be very careful and ensure to differentiate between posing a challenge to him and being a snob.

When you show him, you have a life without him and that he needs to put in some extra efforts to totally win you then you are obviously creating a need for him, the need to get you by all means.

Make him need you by giving him the impression that you accept him for who he is and his weird habits. It's a natural attitude for women to pick on their men, but sometimes it is better you restrain yourself from making that nasty remark about his favorite shirt.

Let Him Know What He Is Missing

Show him what he is missing. Don't be too available for him. Generally, human beings are known to appreciate things more when they are unable to access them.

This also applies to men. Let him know you are good to be with and hard to live without. Just make sure he sees only the happy side of you and don't ever let him make you get upset.

When he realizes what he is truly missing, he will find ways to come around. It is often clear that most guys fall in love when they miss you.

Play A Bit Of Hard To Get

A little hard to get is not a bad idea when you are trying to awaken the commitment instinct in him. If the "hard to get" game doesn't seem to work out because he is already going out with other women, then all you need to do is take things to another level.

You can get this done by going out on dates with other guys. With this, you can surely confirm if he is serious about you and also know if he truly cares about you. If he doesn't seem to care then it's all up to you to determine if he is really worth it.

Contact an Expert

So, if you really want to make your man fall in love with you to ignite the commitment instinct in him, then maybe its high time you swallowed that pride and go out to get some good advice.

There are numerous women who often make mistakes when trying to impress their man. Seeking the assistance of a professional will help you learn from their mistake and prevent you from falling into the same trap.

When you are seeking the assistance of an expert, it will be much better to use the service of someone you know and can create a personal relationship with.

With this, the expert will helpfully give you the chance to deal with your case on a personal level other than making the general approach because all guys are not the same.

You need to understand what makes a mall fall in love and stays in love. No one is perfect but if you truly love your man, you will willingly accept them and their flaws.

Be His Dependent

By making him feel and know that you are someone he can rely on, talk to and share minds with will make him fall in love with you. Give him the freedom to tell you anything with no fear of being judged.

This is the right time to learn how to listen. Give him the free will of talking about his job or even his favorite golf team. You won't find it boring when he talks to you about things he's interested in if you truly care about him.

You are supposed to be his pillar and sanctuary. Trust me he will start needing you more than anything else in this world. Apply all these tips and watch as his commitment instinct is triggered.

WHY WE CHEAT

We are somewhat different from you when it comes to cheating, and a lot of that difference arises from the fact that we tend to define infidelity rather loosely. The truth is if a man wants to cheat he will.

We don't ever need an excuse not to cheat nor will the biggest butt, longest hair or prettiest face persuade us to be faithful. You must've even heard us defend polygamy as something in their genetics trait.

Most we cheat because we are weak, it makes a weak-minded man feel he has power over his woman, It makes him feel he is worth more than her. Most of us think if we cheat on a loyal woman, she will care about him more.

Yes, initially she will be shocked his man has the audacity to cheat on her, especially with a woman who isnt worth it.

Here are some of the reasons why we cheat

We cheat because we are weak

• We are incredibly weak, the truth is we may be physically strong, but we're mentally weak. We have little self-control especially when it comes to women. It's as if there is a switch being flipped every time blood circulation shifts to the secondary "head."

A man cheats when his made to feel inadequate

• A man will indulge in cheating when he feels inadequate.

When a man is repeatedly made to feel like he is less than by their spouse, he seeks to find someone that makes him feel like a priority. In essence, we try to fill the void that our partners used to occupy.

Choice is one of the reasons we cheat

• Nothing "makes" us cheat on our partners, except because we simply choose to. Cheating is a choice, we will either choose to do it, or choose not to. Cheating is the manifestation of unresolved issues not dealt with, a void that is unfulfilled, and the inability to fully commit to the relationship and our partners.

Selfishness

• When most men are caught cheating thy give different excuses. but underneath all those reasons and others it is pretty simple, SELFISHNESS. A selfishness that trumps commitment, integrity of character and honoring another above self.

Due to lack of appreciation

• Some men may feel devalued if their partners don't talk with them, spend time with them, or participate in hobbies with them. Others may feel devalued if their partners stop having regular sex with them.

Or if their partners seem too busy with life, household, children, work, etc to prioritize them. But underlying all of that is a sense that the man does not matter, that he is not valued, and that his partner no longer appreciates him.

This causes the men to seek attention elsewhere, and again in my experience most often it is first this seeking of attention from another. So if you don't prioritize your man, and don't make him feel valued, then you shouldn't be surprised when he seeks attention elsewhere.

While there are numerous stated reasons, one theme that runs through them for men is lack of appreciation and attention. Many men feel they work hard for their families, they internalize their emotions, can feel they have been doing much and not receiving enough in return.

The affair offers the opportunity to receive admiration, approval, new attention, seeing themselves anew in someone else's eyes.

Most men cheat based on the desire for adventure
• The way to escape from the routine and blandness of everyday life. The life between work, boring weekends with kids, in front of the TV set, or computer. The way out from responsibilities, duties, and the specific role we have been given or adopted for ourselves.

When a man feels lack of intimacy and admiration from his spoice he tends to cheat
• Cheating is a result of lack of intimacy in a marriage. Intimacy can be a challenge, but if a man is not feeling fully "seen" in his relationship, or not communicating his needs, it can leave him feeling empty, lonely, angry, and unappreciated.

He may then want to fulfill that need outside the relationship. It's his way of saying "someone else sees me and my value, and understands my needs, so I'm going to get what I need and want there instead". When a man looks outside the relationship for companionship; it's a perceived lack on the man's part of admiration and approval by his partner.

Men tend to base their sense of self on how the people in the room view them; the outside world serves as a mirror of self-worth. So if a man encounters disapproval, disdain, or disappointment at home, they internalize those emotions.

So when a person outside the relationship then provides a counter to those feelings, shows a different "reflection" to the man, the man is often drawn to that. And seeing yourself in an encouraging light, well, that's often very hard to resist.

Most times when a man want out he tends to cheat
• He is looking to end his current relationship and is using external sexual and romantic activities to give his wife or girlfriend "the message" without having to be direct. Or, if he is a man who doesn't like being alone, period, then finding a new and "better" person before leaving a current relationship provides a safer and softer landing.

We cheat due to unreasonable expectations
• Most of us believe that our spouse should meet our every sexual and emotional need, 24/7, without fail. In our narcissistic and self-focused way, we don't understand that our spouse may be juggling multiple priorities (kids, work, home, finances) in addition to us and the relationship.

When she inevitably fails us (in our view), we feel entitled to seek intimate attention elsewhere. But note that we might list millios of reasons why we cheat the truth is we are bound to cheat its in our DNA.

WHY DO WE LOSE INTERESTS IN A RELATIONSHIP?

Men are found to love the chase. We get a rush any time a new woman finds us attractive, funny, smart, and irresistible. We do everything we can just to prove to ourselves that we can get the girl.

But once she shows interest and we actually gets her, we don't have anything to prove anymore. Our fear of commitment kicks in and our first instinct is to run. So, we move onto the next conquest so we can get that ego boost again by pursuing someone new.

Men who need the ego boost of a new conquest are insecure. We lose interest when a girl shows interest because on some level we feel unworthy. We need to go chase after another girl to feel worthy again.

Men can often be difficult creatures for women to understand. The slow brush off or the fade away seems to be much more common today than in the past.

The truth is, sometimes it's just easier for men to fade to black and stop returning your calls rather than being honest with you about why they have lost interest in you.

Here are some of the reasons why we lose intesrests in relationship

We lose interest when a woman is boring

- If you don't have much to say, and if you don't have too many interesting thoughts and observations to share, and you don't know how to respond to what the guy you are seeing says, thinks and believes in, you are not going to keep a great guy's interest for very long.

Boring dates feel like a torture, and no one is interested in going into one or sticking around when they realize that they have to push the conversation to simply fill the time.

Surely there is no shortcut to becoming a more interesting person, but there is a great, long-term solution you start to learn more things about yourself, about your environment and the world.

TV, magazines, books, meeting new people, watching different shows, and engaging in social events will give you much more material to think about and form your views on.

Surely, there is a lot of junk out there on TV and in magazines, but there is also lots of good material. It is your duty to choose and "filter" the bad stuff out.

We tend to lose interest in a relationship when our spouse takes feminity too far

- While equality and equal rights are great, more and more women take the notion of feminism way too far. For some women showing and proving to the world that they can do and be anything a guy can is their life's mission.

Equal opportunities for women is a great concept

without which no society has the right to call itself free and civilized.

However, when this equality comes at the expense of femininity and elegance women pay a high price of becoming very unattractive to the opposite sex.

It's a fundamental law of nature that masculine, confident, attractive men are attracted to the opposite feminine women, women who possess a feminine voice, walk, and manners.

The fact is no one would ever suggest that a woman should stay home and cook and clean. This is not what it is about.

A woman can be very educated, successful and independent and still retain her femininity and be proud of being a woman and stop hiding the fact that you are different from guys. You are and it's good news.

Men lose intrests in relationship if his spouse is not good in bed

- Many women either ruin the romantic tension and the connection with the guy in bed. Few women act in a way that will make sleeping with them a great, memorable experience that the guy is eager to repeat.

Some of the big turn-offs for guys are women who are either too quiet in bed (not making any sounds that would indicate their enjoyment and would look like they are bored), or those who talk too much, or say something inappropriate and irrelevant at the very wrong time.

when a woman talks too much men tend to lose interest

- No matter how smart or cool a woman is if she talks too much and tend to dominate the conversation or interrupt all the time she would get feeling out of place or he would be bored because there is no room for him to say any thing.

Men lose intesrest in relationship when a woman is too feisty

- When a woman challenges her partner for a reason or no reason just for the sake of showing to him over and over that her man cannot control her. She will disagree on the place to eat, go out at, travel to, and do not because she doesn't like his idea, but because she wants to demonstrate to him that he cannot control her.

A strong, confident guy will be turned-off and will lose interest in such a woman quickly because to him such an attitude is incompatible with a very notion of being feminine. These reason maks most men lose interest in the relationship.

The truth is, No one can correctly state to any woman why a man loses interest in her because circumstances and situations differ.

However, by paying attention to the above possible issues listed that you might be having in your interactions with guys, you will surely improve the chances of keeping any guy's interest and coming across as a more attractive and desirable woman.

HOW TO AVOID REJECTION FROM MEN

Rejection is the most terrifying and absolutely the worst thing that could really happen to you. You get a man who after a couple days or dates, he decides to ignores you.

Feeling rejected leads to trauma and for some people it makes it had for them to want to meet new people or try new relationship out due to their past experience.

Here are some of the things to consider so as to avoid being rejected from men

Don't be too available

- When you are not too available and and the same time not too distanced your man would want more if you. Not doing anything 24 hours and being available all the time can cause rejection try and make a big deal out of planning a short holiday away with the girls.

He will begin to miss you before you have even parted! Then while you are away, keep in touch, but make it brief.

Don't give away too many details about what you have been doing, let his imagination do the talking, and feed it with sexual tit-bits to get his sexual desire for you. Tell him how much you miss his kisses and cuddles, that sort of thing.

Soon you will notice that his texts get a little bit soppier because he is missing you. When it is finally time to come home, he will be all over you, because of all the anticipation you have built up.

Change something radical about yourself

- A man wants something new, refreshed, something he hasn't seen you do before. If you do things that cause him to take a second look at you now and then, the chances of being rejected by you man is low.

For example, a man is more likely to notice and feel attracted to a change in your appearance if it is obviously different to your usual look. Change is exciting because it is new and it makes him feel like he has discovered a new facet of your personality.

If you want a change and you want to take advantage of the chance to grab his attention while you're at it, drastically change your hair colour and you will feel and act like a different person.

He'll immediately sense the sexy difference in your personality, and the sexy confidence, and be turned on by the sexual implication of dating, let's say, a redhead. If you don't want to go as far as a permanent change then look to your wardrobe and put together a sexy new look. Some noticeably high heels should do the trick if you normally wear flats.

Try and encourage attention from other men

- This is less about making your man jealous, and more about making him feel good. Suggesting that a woman should encourage attention from other men, doesn't mean make your own man feel insecure.

It just means using the opportunity to show him you're his, and you will make him feel proud. All men have a primal instinct to compete against each other, especially when it comes to women.

If he knows he's got the woman all the other guys are ogling, his ego will be swelling. Guys always seem to be a lot more clingy and affectionate too when they know there are half a dozen other men showing interest in their woman.

Be reserved

- Less is always more. When you give a guy everything on a plate, there is no challenge, no mystery and he would feel he has known all about you to act up but when you don't spill it all out he would want to know more. This applies to your everyday conversation.

You don't have to give him all the nitty gritty details of your day or your night out. That is what your girlfriends are for. Even if he asks, don't be tempted to go into detail.

Give minimal information and he will make the effort to probe you for more. That's when you know you've got his full attention, and he is more likely to actually be interested in what you do tell him because he is specifically digging for the information,

The less you tell him about your life, the more he will thinking about you and wondering about what you are doing. Before you know it, you will be all he thinks about.

Inspire your man

- What makes you irreplaceable in the eyes of your man? Your ability to reach deep into the depths of who he is and inspire him. To put it more bluntly, you must offer something that is much rarer and valuable than sex if you want to avoid being rejected .

Ask yourself:

what are you bringing to the table beside a physical hookup that he values deeply? Sex is readily available. Having it isn't enough to make a relationship and withholding it isn't enough to cast some kind of "love spell" on a guy to stay or to avoid you.

We have a deep unconscious fear that our lives, our contribution to the world and our existence is pointless, meaningless, and insignificant. At the same time, every man has hopes, dreams, and aspirations, and here's the major lesson.

In order for a man to feel truly alive and truly fulfilled, he needs to be pursuing his deepest aspiration and his "mission" in life.

Your ultimate gift as a woman is to inspire him to do that, to realize his ultimate potential as a man. No man would ever reject such a woman or otherwise he still doest know what he wants in life.

CONCLUSION

Isn't it hard to know what we guys really want in you? Do we just want sex or do we want to really fall in love? Why is it so hard to make us commit? What are we afraid of? Guys are a mystery until you discover what we really want in you ladies.

Part of the problem is that we don't know what we want ourselves until the right woman comes along. If you asked a single guy what he wanted in a woman, the answer would be painfully simplistic and revolve around sex.

If you took his word at face value, you would think you had to spend a fortune on breast implants and plastic surgery in order to give a man what he wants.

Save your money. Use it to buy yourself clothes that reflect your personality. We end up going for the girls who have unique aura about them, who are self-confident and intriguing looking. There's something about a girl that has that aura of confidence that makes us think beyond sex and want to get to know the person behind the body.

Being self confident isn't the same thing as being stand-offish. Truly confident people are always interested in others. When a cute guy approaches you, you don't need to pretend like you're not interested. The fact that you are interested in him will give him the courage to pursue you. The fact that you're not interested in him exclusively will make him feel like he has to work for you.

What we really want is a woman who makes us feel the confidence and self-respect that is lacking in our own lives. We want to be admired and appreciated, but we also want our partners to be admired and appreciated as well.

What we want is mutual respect. That's why, if a guy has to

choose between a girl with a great body and a girl with a great mind and personality as a life partner, he'll choose the latter.

MY GIFT TO YOU CLICK THE LINK BELOW

https://nowthis.life/rac/

PLEASE WRITE A REVIEW!

If this book helped you out in anyway, please
help me to help others by writing a review!

CLICK HERE TO LEAVE A REVIEW

Still, if you did not get anything new from this book
or you were not impacted in some way, I would still like
to hear what you have to say. Either way, I will know what
am doing right or wrong and to improve in the future. I
wouldn't like to take your money and not deliver. So please,
take just 2 minutes to let me know what you think.

Everyone is searching for help on how to improve their
lives for the better and one thing they do look for are reviews.
If this book has a lot amazing reviews with great comments,
they will buy the book and read it and so the ripples effects
of goodness spreads. But if it doesn't have any great reviews
and comments, they don't buy the book and read it.

I know this book can positively impact and help
someone and you can help that person by writing
your thoughts and takeaways from the book.

Additionally, I would like to read your review and hear how
this book has helped you in anyway at shape or form. My plan is
to print every single review and hang them on my home office
wall to read for inspiration and motivation throughout the day.

Your great review helps me personally to stay focused
and be able to validate all the hard work and lots of
hours invested in preparing this book for you.

CLICK THE LINK TO LEAVE A REVIEW

Thank you again for reading this book and all of your support, I am truly honored and grateful to have been of help. I look forward to helping you make this year the best ever for you and your family!

HTTPS://NOWTHIS.LIFE/RAC/